Let's Chill: CBD Essentials for Beginners

Chapter 1: Introduction to CBD

What is CBD?

A Brief History of Cannabis

Different Types of Cannabinoids

Legal Status of CBD

Chapter 2: How CBD Works

The Endocannabinoid System (ECS)

CBD and Receptors

CBD's Mechanisms of Action

Chapter 3: Types of CBD Products

CBD Oil and Tinctures

CBD Capsules and Softgels

CBD Edibles

CBD Topicals

CBD Vapes and Inhalables

Appendices

Glossary of CBD Terminology

Quick Reference Guide for CBD Dosage

State and International CBD Regulations

Sources of Reliable Information on CBD

Chapter 1: Introduction to CBD

What is CBD?

Section 1.1: Defining CBD

Cannabidiol, or CBD, is a natural compound found in the Cannabis sativa plant. It belongs to a class of compounds known as **cannabinoids**. While CBD is just one of over a hundred different cannabinoids identified in cannabis, it has garnered significant attention for its potential therapeutic properties and its lack of intoxicating effects.

Section 1.2: A Brief History of Cannabis

The use of cannabis dates back thousands of years, with historical records showing its cultivation for medicinal and industrial purposes in various cultures around the world. Cannabis was used for pain relief, as an anesthetic, and for its psychoactive properties, long before modern science understood the compounds responsible for these effects.

Section 1.3: Different Types of Cannabinoids

Cannabinoids are the chemical compounds responsible for the unique effects of cannabis. Two of the most well-known cannabinoids are **CBD (cannabidiol) and THC (tetrahydrocannabinol).**

CBD (Cannabidiol): CBD is non-psychoactive, meaning it does not produce the "high" associated with cannabis use. Instead, it's known for its potential therapeutic benefits, including pain relief, anxiety reduction, and more.

THC (Tetrahydrocannabinol): THC is the primary psychoactive cannabinoid in cannabis. It's responsible for the euphoria or "high" that many people associate with marijuana use.

Section 1.4: Legal Status of CBD

The legal status of CBD varies from one region to another. In some places, CBD extracted from hemp plants (a variety of cannabis with low THC content) is legal and widely available. In others, CBD derived from marijuana plants may be subject to stricter regulations due to its higher THC content.

Section 1.5: CBD in Modern Wellness

In recent years, CBD has experienced a surge in popularity, particularly in the wellness and health industries. People are turning to CBD for a variety of potential health benefits, often seeking natural alternatives to traditional medications.

Section 1.6: Objectives of This Book

In this book, we aim to provide a comprehensive understanding of CBD, its potential benefits, and its various applications. We will explore the science behind how CBD works in the body, the different types of CBD products available, and the potential advantages and risks associated with its use. Additionally, we will discuss CBD's legal status, offer practical guidance on incorporating it into your wellness routine, and explore its future in healthcare.

Whether you are considering using CBD for a specific health concern, are curious about its effects, or want to stay informed about this rapidly evolving field, this book will serve as a valuable resource on your journey to understanding CBD and its potential impact on your well-being.

In the following chapters, we will delve deeper into the science of how CBD interacts with the body's endocannabinoid system, explore the various forms of CBD products, and discuss the specific benefits of CBD for both physical and mental health.

A Brief History of Cannabis

Section 1.2: A Brief History of Cannabis

Cannabis, one of the world's oldest cultivated plants, has a rich history deeply intertwined with human civilization. Its story spans thousands of years and diverse cultures, revealing a complex tapestry of uses and perceptions.

Ancient Beginnings

The history of cannabis cultivation dates back as far as 5000 BCE in what is now modern-day Taiwan, where archaeologists have discovered the remnants of hemp cord in pottery. It is believed that cannabis originated in Central Asia and gradually spread to various parts of the world, becoming an integral part of many ancient cultures.

Early Medicinal Use

Cannabis was initially used for its medicinal properties. Ancient Chinese texts from around 2700 BCE describe its use as a treatment for various ailments, including pain and digestive disorders. Cannabis was also used in ancient India, where it played a role in the Ayurvedic system of medicine.

Spiritual and Religious Significance

In India, cannabis assumed spiritual significance, with references to it found in sacred texts like the Vedas. It was associated with Lord Shiva, one of the principal deities in Hinduism, and was considered a divine plant that facilitated communication with the gods.

Spread Across Continents

As civilizations and trade routes expanded, so did the use of cannabis. It spread throughout Asia, the Middle East, and Africa. In the Middle East, it was used for its psychoactive properties and for its fiber to make textiles and ropes.

Introduction to the Western World

Cannabis made its way to the Western world in various forms. It was used for medicinal purposes in Europe during the Middle Ages and was even cultivated in early American colonies for its fiber.

Recreational Use and Prohibition

In the 19th century, cannabis began to be used recreationally in the West. However, as concerns about its psychoactive effects grew, especially in the early 20th century, several countries began implementing restrictions and prohibitions on its use.

The 20th Century and the War on Drugs

The 20th century saw the global push for cannabis prohibition, driven largely by political and cultural factors. In the United States, the Marihuana Tax Act of 1937 effectively banned cannabis use and cultivation. This was followed by a stricter approach in the 1970s with the Controlled Substances Act, which classified cannabis as a Schedule I drug.

Changing Attitudes and Legalization

Despite decades of prohibition, attitudes toward cannabis began to shift in the late 20th century. The emergence of the medical marijuana movement in the 1990s paved the way for the legalization of cannabis for medical use in several U.S. states. In the 21st century, several countries and U.S. states have moved toward full legalization for both medical and recreational use.

Today, cannabis is experiencing resurgence in interest for its potential medical and therapeutic applications. It is also being explored for its industrial uses, including the production of hemp-based products such as textiles, paper, and food products.

As we move forward in this book, we will delve deeper into the specific compound found within cannabis, cannabidiol (CBD), and its potential benefits and uses in modern wellness and healthcare.

Different Types of Cannabinoids

Section 1.3: Different Types of Cannabinoids

Cannabinoids are a diverse group of chemical compounds found in the Cannabis sativa plant. Each type of cannabinoid interacts with the human body's endocannabinoid system in its unique way, resulting in a wide range of effects. While there are over 100 known cannabinoids, we'll focus on some of the most well-known and studied ones, including:

1. CBD (Cannabidiol):

- **Properties:** CBD is non-psychoactive, meaning it doesn't produce the euphoric "high" associated with cannabis use. It's known for its potential therapeutic benefits, including pain relief, anxiety reduction, and anti-inflammatory properties.
- **Research:** CBD has been studied extensively for various medical conditions, and the FDA has approved a CBD-based prescription medication called Epidiolex for certain types of epilepsy.

2. THC (Tetrahydrocannabinol):

- **Properties:** THC is the primary psychoactive compound in cannabis, responsible for the mind-altering effects often associated with marijuana use. It can induce feelings of euphoria, relaxation, and altered perception of time and space.
- **Medical Uses:** THC has been used medically for its pain-relieving properties and as an appetite stimulant in conditions like cancer and AIDS. However, its psychoactive effects can limit its medical applications.

3. CBG (Cannabigerol):

- **Properties:** Often referred to as the **"mother cannabinoid,"** CBG is a non-psychoactive compound that can be found in higher concentrations in the early stages of cannabis growth. It's considered a precursor to other cannabinoids.
- **Research:** Although research on CBG is in its early stages, it shows potential for various therapeutic applications, including as an anti-inflammatory, pain reliever, and potential treatment for glaucoma.

4. CBN (Cannabinol):

- **Properties: CBN** is a mildly psychoactive cannabinoid that results from the degradation of THC. It's often associated with sedative effects and is believed to contribute to the "couch-lock" sensation sometimes experienced with certain cannabis strains.
- **Research:** Research into CBN is limited, but it's been studied for its potential as a sleep aid and for its antibacterial properties.

5. CBC (Cannabichromene):

- **Properties: CBC** is a non-psychoactive cannabinoid that's found in trace amounts in cannabis. It's thought to work synergistically with other cannabinoids and is often present in full-spectrum CBD products.
- **Research:** Although research on CBC is ongoing, it's been studied for its potential anti-inflammatory, pain-relieving, and neuroprotective effects.

6. THCV (Tetrahydrocannabivarin):

- **Properties: THCV** is a cannabinoid with varying effects depending on the dose. At low doses, it may act as an appetite suppressant, while at higher doses, it can produce effects similar to THC, though typically of shorter duration.

- **Research:** Research on THCV is limited but suggests potential applications for weight management and diabetes control.

These are just a few of the many cannabinoids present in cannabis. Each one has its unique characteristics, and researchers continue to explore their potential therapeutic benefits. Understanding the diversity of cannabinoids is crucial for comprehending the various effects and potential medical applications of cannabis and its derivatives.

In the following chapters, we will dive deeper into the specific benefits of CBD, THC, and other cannabinoids, as well as their interactions with the body's endocannabinoid system.

Legal Status of CBD

Section 1.4: The Evolution of CBD's Legal Status

The legal status of CBD (cannabidiol) has undergone significant changes over the decades, reflecting evolving attitudes and scientific understanding of this compound. This section provides a detailed overview of the changing legal landscape of CBD, both at the federal and state levels.

1930s to 1990s: Cannabis Prohibition Era

- **Marihuana Tax Act (1937):** The Marihuana Tax Act effectively banned the use and cultivation of cannabis in the United States. This marked the beginning of the era of cannabis prohibition.
- **Controlled Substances Act (1970):** Cannabis, including CBD, was classified as a Schedule I controlled substance under the Controlled Substances Act of 1970, placing it in the same category as drugs like heroin and LSD.

1990s to Early 2000s: Emergence of Medical Marijuana

- **California's Proposition 215 (1996):** California became the first U.S. state to legalize medical marijuana, setting a precedent for other states to follow.
- **Federal Response:** Despite state-level initiatives, federal law continued to classify cannabis, including CBD, as illegal. This created tension between state and federal laws.

2014 to 2018: Farm Bill and Hemp Legalization

- **Farm Bill (2014):** The 2014 Farm Bill allowed for the cultivation of industrial hemp for research purposes by institutions of higher education and state departments of agriculture. This marked a significant step towards distinguishing hemp (low in THC and high in CBD) from marijuana.
- **Farm Bill (2018):** The 2018 Farm Bill was a major milestone in CBD's legal journey. It removed hemp and its derivatives, including CBD, from the list of controlled substances. This effectively legalized the cultivation, production, and sale of hemp-derived CBD at the federal level.

Current Status: Federal and State Laws

- **Federal Level:** Hemp-derived CBD (with less than 0.3% THC) is legal under federal law. It can be sold, purchased, and used throughout the United States. The FDA regulates CBD products intended for human consumption and prohibits making health claims without FDA approval.
- **State Level:** States have the authority to establish their own CBD laws, which can vary widely. While hemp-derived CBD is legal in most states, the legality of CBD derived from marijuana (higher in THC) varies depending on state laws.

States Where CBD Is Legal (Hemp-Derived):

- As of my knowledge cutoff date in September 2021, hemp-derived CBD is generally legal in most U.S. states, including but not limited to California, New York, Texas, Florida, and Colorado.

States with Restrictions or Specific Laws:

- Some states have implemented specific regulations related to CBD products, such as labeling requirements or restrictions on the sale of CBD-infused foods and beverages.

States Where CBD Is Illegal:

- In some states, CBD laws are more restrictive, and the sale and use of CBD products may be prohibited or allowed only in limited circumstances.
- It's important to note that CBD's legal status can change, so it's crucial to stay informed about the specific laws and regulations in your state. Additionally, while hemp-derived CBD is legal under federal law, products must comply with FDA regulations, and quality control is essential to ensure the safety and potency of CBD products.

For the most up-to-date information on CBD's legal status in your state, it's advisable to consult your state's official government website or a legal professional familiar with your local laws. Additionally, keep in mind that developments in CBD's legal status may have occurred after my last knowledge update in September 2021.

Chapter 2: How CBD Works

The Endocannabinoid System (ECS)

Section 2.1: Understanding the Endocannabinoid System (ECS)

To comprehend how CBD works in the body, it's essential to familiarize yourself with the endocannabinoid system (ECS). The ECS is a complex regulatory system present in humans and many animals, which plays a critical role in maintaining various physiological processes.

Section 2.2: Components of the ECS

The ECS consists of three primary components:

1. Endocannabinoids: These are natural compounds produced within the body. The two most well-studied endocannabinoids are anandamide and 2-arachidonoylglycerol (2-AG). These compounds are similar in structure to cannabinoids found in the cannabis plant.

2. Receptors: The ECS has two main types of receptors, known as CB1 and CB2 receptors. CB1 receptors are primarily located in the central nervous system, while CB2 receptors are predominantly found in immune cells and peripheral tissues. These receptors are like locks, and endocannabinoids or cannabinoids act as keys that bind to them.

3. Enzymes: Enzymes play a crucial role in the ECS by breaking down endocannabinoids once they've fulfilled their function. The two key enzymes are fatty acid amide hydrolase (FAAH), which breaks down anandamide, and monoacylglycerol lipase (MAGL), which breaks down 2-AG.

Section 2.3: The Role of the ECS

The **ECS** acts as a homeostatic regulator, helping the body maintain balance or equilibrium in various physiological processes. **It is involved in:**

- **Pain Regulation:** The ECS plays a role in modulating pain perception, both in response to injury and in chronic pain conditions.
- **Inflammation:** It helps regulate the immune response, including the body's inflammatory response.
- **Mood and Stress:** The ECS has an impact on mood, stress response, and anxiety.
- **Appetite and Metabolism:** It can influence appetite and metabolic processes.
- **Sleep:** The ECS is associated with sleep regulation and circadian rhythms.

Section 2.4: How CBD Interacts with the ECS

CBD interacts with the ECS by influencing its receptors, but unlike THC, it does not bind directly to CB1 or CB2 receptors. Instead, it modulates the ECS in more indirect ways.

CBD and CB1 Receptors: CBD can influence CB1 receptors by inhibiting the enzyme FAAH, which normally breaks down anandamide. By inhibiting FAAH, CBD can increase anandamide levels in the body, potentially leading to mood enhancement and pain relief.

CBD and CB2 Receptors: CBD also has an impact on CB2 receptors, which are primarily associated with the immune system. By influencing CB2 receptors, CBD may play a role in reducing inflammation and supporting the immune response.

Section 2.5: Beyond Cannabinoid Receptors

CBD's effects are not limited to cannabinoid receptors. It interacts with various other receptor systems in the body, such as the serotonin receptors (5-HT1A), which are involved in mood regulation. This may explain CBD's potential anti-anxiety and antidepressant effects.

Section 2.6: The Entourage Effect

CBD's effectiveness is often enhanced when it's used alongside other cannabinoids and compounds found in the cannabis plant. This synergy is known as the "entourage effect," where various components work together to produce more significant benefits than they would individually.

Section 2.7: Conclusion

Understanding the ECS is essential to grasp how CBD exerts its potential therapeutic effects. By modulating this intricate system, CBD may help regulate various bodily functions, from pain perception to mood and inflammation. In the following chapters, we'll delve into the specific benefits of CBD and its applications for physical and mental health.

Section 2.8: CBD and Receptors

CBD's effects on the human body are primarily mediated through its interaction with various receptors, particularly those within the endocannabinoid system (ECS). This section delves into how CBD influences these receptors and the resulting physiological responses.

CBD and CB1 Receptors: Indirect Modulation

One of the primary receptor types in the ECS is the CB1 receptor, mainly found in the central nervous system. Unlike THC, which directly binds to CB1 receptors, CBD does not directly activate or bind with them. Instead, it influences CB1 receptors in an indirect manner.

CBD inhibits the action of the enzyme FAAH (fatty acid amide hydrolase), responsible for breaking down anandamide, an endocannabinoid that naturally binds to CB1 receptors. By inhibiting FAAH, CBD prolongs the presence of anandamide in the body, allowing it to exert its effects more effectively. Anandamide is associated with mood regulation, pain perception, and other functions related to the central nervous system.

CBD and CB2 Receptors: Modulating the Immune Response

CB2 receptors are predominantly found in immune cells and peripheral tissues, where they play a crucial role in regulating the immune system's response to inflammation and injury. CBD also interacts with CB2 receptors, albeit in a different way than THC.

CBD's interaction with CB2 receptors may contribute to its potential anti-inflammatory and immunomodulatory effects. By modulating these receptors, CBD can influence the immune response, potentially reducing inflammation and its associated symptoms.

CBD and Non-Cannabinoid Receptors: A Multifaceted Approach

While CBD's interaction with cannabinoid receptors is well-documented, its effects go beyond the ECS. CBD also interacts with several other receptor systems in the body, contributing to its diverse range of potential benefits:

- **Serotonin Receptors (5-HT1A):** CBD activates serotonin receptors, specifically the 5-HT1A receptor subtype. Serotonin is a neurotransmitter associated with mood regulation. By influencing these receptors, CBD may have anxiolytic (anxiety-reducing) and antidepressant effects.
- **Vanilloid Receptors (TRPV1):** CBD can interact with TRPV1 receptors, which are involved in pain perception and inflammation. This interaction may contribute to CBD's potential analgesic (pain-relieving) and anti-inflammatory properties.
- **Adenosine Receptors:** CBD interacts with adenosine receptors, which play a role in regulating various physiological processes, including sleep, inflammation, and cardiovascular function. CBD's influence on these receptors may contribute to its potential calming and anti-inflammatory effects.

CBD and the Entourage Effect

It's important to note that the effects of CBD are often enhanced when it is used alongside other cannabinoids and compounds found in the cannabis plant. This synergy is known as the "entourage effect." When CBD is combined with a spectrum of cannabinoids, terpenes, and other phytochemicals, they can work together to produce more significant and diverse benefits than they would individually.

In summary, CBD's interaction with receptors, both within and beyond the ECS, contributes to its potential therapeutic effects. By modulating these receptors, CBD can influence a wide range of physiological processes, making it a versatile compound with diverse applications for physical and mental well-being.

Section 2.8: CBD's Mechanisms of Action

CBD's diverse range of potential therapeutic effects stems from its ability to interact with various biological systems and receptors in the body. Understanding the mechanisms through which CBD exerts its effects can shed light on its versatility in addressing a wide array of health concerns.

1. Interaction with the Endocannabinoid System (ECS):

The primary mechanism through which CBD exerts its effects is by interacting with the endocannabinoid system (ECS). The ECS is a complex regulatory system composed of three main components: endocannabinoids (like anandamide and 2-AG), receptors (CB1 and CB2), and enzymes (FAAH and MAGL).

- **Inhibition of FAAH:** CBD inhibits the enzyme FAAH, which normally breaks down anandamide, a naturally occurring endocannabinoid. By inhibiting FAAH, CBD increases anandamide levels in the body. Anandamide is associated with mood regulation, pain perception, and other functions related to the central nervous system.
- **Modulation of CB1 and CB2 Receptors:** While CBD does not directly bind to CB1 and CB2 receptors as THC does, it influences these receptors indirectly. CBD's interaction with CB1 and CB2 receptors contributes to its potential therapeutic effects on pain, inflammation, mood, and immune function.

2. Serotonin Receptors (5-HT1A):

CBD's interaction with serotonin receptors, specifically the 5-HT1A receptor subtype, plays a role in its potential anxiolytic (anxiety-reducing) and antidepressant effects. Serotonin is a neurotransmitter associated with mood regulation. By activating these receptors, CBD may help modulate mood and reduce symptoms of anxiety and depression.

3. Vanilloid Receptors (TRPV1):

CBD interacts with TRPV1 receptors, which are part of the vanilloid receptor family. These receptors are involved in pain perception and the regulation of body temperature. CBD's interaction with TRPV1 receptors may contribute to its potential analgesic (pain-relieving) and anti-inflammatory effects.

4. Adenosine Receptors:

CBD interacts with adenosine receptors, particularly the A2A receptor subtype. Adenosine receptors play a role in regulating various physiological processes, including sleep, inflammation, and cardiovascular function. CBD's influence on these receptors may contribute to its potential calming effects, support for sleep, and anti-inflammatory properties.

5. GPR55 Receptors:

CBD has been found to modulate GPR55 receptors, which are involved in regulating blood pressure and bone density. By interacting with GPR55 receptors, CBD may contribute to its potential cardiovascular benefits and influence bone health.

6. PPARγ Receptors:

CBD can activate peroxisome proliferator-activated receptor-gamma (PPARγ) receptors, which are involved in metabolic regulation, inflammation, and cell differentiation. CBD's interaction with PPARγ receptors may have implications for its potential benefits in metabolic disorders and inflammatory conditions.

7. Non-Receptor-Mediated Pathways:

CBD's mechanisms of action are not solely reliant on receptor interactions. It can also influence various signaling pathways, ion channels, and enzymes, which can contribute to its broad range of effects.

In summary, CBD exerts its effects through a complex interplay of mechanisms involving the ECS, serotonin receptors, vanilloid receptors, adenosine receptors, and more. This multifaceted approach to modulating physiological processes makes CBD a versatile compound with potential applications in a wide array of health conditions. However, it's important to note that research on CBD's mechanisms of action is ongoing, and our understanding of its full range of effects continues to evolve.

Chapter 3: Types of CBD Products

Section 2.9: Introduction to CBD Oil and Tinctures

CBD oil and tinctures are among the most popular and versatile forms of CBD products available. They offer a convenient way to incorporate CBD into your daily wellness routine. In this chapter, we will explore the characteristics, benefits, and considerations of CBD oil and tinctures in great detail.

Section 3.0: What Is CBD Oil and What Are Tinctures?

CBD Oil:

Ingredients: CBD oil typically consists of CBD extract (either from hemp or marijuana) and a carrier oil, such as coconut oil, hemp seed oil, or MCT oil. The carrier oil is used to dilute the CBD extract for easy consumption.

Tinctures:

Ingredients: Tinctures are similar to CBD oil but are alcohol-based. They contain CBD extract, an alcohol base (commonly ethanol), and sometimes additional flavorings.

Section 3.1: How CBD Oil and Tinctures Are Made

Extraction Methods:

- CBD extract is obtained from the hemp or marijuana plant through various extraction methods, such as CO2 extraction or ethanol extraction. These methods separate CBD and other cannabinoids from the plant material.

Carrier Oils:

- The CBD extract is then mixed with a carrier oil to create CBD oil. This dilution is essential for accurate dosing and to make the CBD more palatable.

Section 3.2: Potency and Concentration

CBD oil and tinctures come in various concentrations, usually measured in milligrams (mg) of CBD per milliliter (ml) of product. Higher concentrations are suitable for those who require larger doses or have specific health concerns. Beginners may opt for lower concentrations to start with.

Section 3.3: Administration Methods

CBD oil and tinctures offer flexibility in terms of how they can be consumed:

- **Sublingual:** This method involves placing a few drops of CBD oil or tincture under the tongue and holding it there for a minute or two before swallowing. Sublingual administration allows for quick absorption through the mucous membranes, resulting in faster onset of effects.
- **Incorporating into Food and Beverages:** You can mix CBD oil or tincture into your favorite foods or beverages. Keep in mind that the onset of effects may be slower compared to the sublingual method because the CBD must pass through the digestive system.

- **Topical Application**: Some CBD tinctures are formulated for topical use. These are applied directly to the skin, where they can potentially provide localized relief for issues like pain or skin conditions.

Section 3.4: Benefits of CBD Oil and Tinctures

- **Precise Dosage:** CBD oil and tinctures allow for precise dosing, making it easier to tailor your CBD intake to your specific needs.
- **Quick Onset:** Sublingual administration provides a faster onset of effects compared to other consumption methods.
- **Versatility:** You can use CBD oil and tinctures in various ways, making them suitable for different preferences and lifestyles.

Section 3.5: Considerations and Tips

- **Quality Matters:** Choose products from reputable manufacturers that provide third-party lab testing results to ensure product quality and CBD content.
- **Start Low and Go Slow:** If you're new to CBD, start with a low dose and gradually increase it until you achieve the desired effects.
- **Consult a Healthcare Professional:** If you're taking medications or have underlying health conditions, consult a healthcare provider before using CBD products to avoid potential interactions.

Section 3.6: Conclusion

CBD oil and tinctures offer a convenient and versatile way to incorporate CBD into your wellness routine. Their precise dosing and quick onset of effects make them popular choices for individuals seeking the potential benefits of CBD. In the following chapters, we will explore other types of CBD products, their benefits, and considerations for use.

Chapter 3 provides a detailed overview of CBD oil and tinctures, including their composition, manufacturing processes, administration methods, benefits, and important considerations for consumers.

CBD Capsules and Softgels

Section 3.7: CBD Capsules and Softgels

In this section, we will explore CBD capsules and softgels, another popular and convenient form of CBD product. These solid, pre-measured doses offer specific advantages for users seeking precise dosing and ease of consumption.

Section 3.7.1: Introduction to CBD Capsules and Softgels

CBD Capsules:

- **Composition:** CBD capsules contain a measured dose of CBD extract enclosed within a gelatin or vegetarian capsule shell.
- **Benefits:** Capsules offer accurate dosing and convenience. They are tasteless, odorless, and easy to swallow.

CBD Softgels:

- **Composition:** CBD softgels are similar to capsules but use a gel-like casing that is often easier to swallow and may dissolve faster.
- **Benefits:** Softgels offer the same advantages as capsules, with the added benefit of quicker absorption due to their faster dissolution in the digestive tract.

Section 3.7.2: How CBD Capsules and Softgels Are Made

- **CBD Extract:** The CBD extract used in capsules and softgels is typically derived from hemp plants through various extraction methods, ensuring high purity and consistency.
- **Precise Dosing:** The manufacturing process ensures that each capsule or softgel contains an exact amount of CBD, making it easy for users to monitor their CBD intake accurately.

Section 3.7.3: Potency and Concentration

Like other CBD products, capsules and softgels come in a range of concentrations, allowing users to choose a strength that aligns with their specific needs and preferences.

Section 3.7.4: Administration Method

- **Oral Consumption:** CBD capsules and softgels are ingested orally. They pass through the digestive system, and the CBD is absorbed in the gastrointestinal tract, resulting in a slower onset of effects compared to sublingual methods.

Section 3.7.5: Benefits of CBD Capsules and Softgels

- **Precise Dosage:** Capsules and softgels provide a consistent and exact CBD dosage, making it easy to track your daily intake.
- **Discreet and Convenient:** These forms of CBD are discreet and convenient for on-the-go use, as there's no need for measuring or mixing.
- **Tasteless and Odorless:** They are ideal for users who want to avoid the taste of CBD oil or tinctures.

Section 3.7.6: Considerations and Tips

- **Digestive Absorption:** Keep in mind that the onset of effects with capsules and softgels is typically slower than with sublingual methods due to digestive processing.
- **Purity and Quality:** Choose products from reputable manufacturers with third-party lab testing to ensure purity and CBD content.
- **Allergies and Dietary Restrictions:** Check the ingredients list, especially if you have dietary restrictions or allergies, as some capsules may contain additional components like gelatin or additives.

Section 3.7.7: Conclusion

CBD capsules and softgels offer an easy and precise way to incorporate CBD into your daily routine. They are favored by individuals who prefer standardized dosing and the convenience of a pre-measured format. In the following chapters, we will explore other types of CBD products, their benefits, and considerations for use.

Chapter 3 provides a detailed overview of CBD capsules and softgels, including their composition, manufacturing processes, dosing, administration methods, benefits, and important considerations for consumers.

CBD Edibles

Section 3.7.8: CBD Edibles

CBD edibles are a popular and enjoyable way to incorporate cannabidiol into your daily routine. In this section, we will explore the world of CBD-infused edibles, discussing their characteristics, benefits, and considerations for consumers.

Section 3.7.9: Introduction to CBD Edibles

What Are CBD Edibles?

- CBD edibles are food products that have been infused with CBD extract, typically derived from hemp. These can include gummies, chocolates, beverages, and more.

Taste and Variety:

- CBD edibles come in various flavors and forms, making them an enjoyable way to consume CBD, especially for those who dislike the natural taste of CBD oil.

Section 3.8: How CBD Edibles Are Made

CBD Extract:

- High-quality CBD extract from hemp plants is used to infuse edibles. The extract is carefully processed to remove any unwanted compounds and ensure consistency.

Food Preparation:

- The CBD extract is added to the edible product during the manufacturing process. This can involve baking, mixing, or otherwise incorporating the extract into the food.

Section 3.8.1: Potency and Dosage

Standardized Dosing:

- CBD edibles provide a convenient way to achieve standardized dosing since each edible typically contains a specific amount of CBD. This makes it easy to monitor your CBD intake accurately.

Onset of Effects:

- The onset of effects with edibles is generally slower compared to sublingual methods, as the CBD must first pass through the digestive system. Effects can typically be felt within 30 minutes to 2 hours after consumption.

Section 3.8.2: Administration Method

Oral Consumption:

- CBD edibles are consumed orally and are absorbed through the digestive tract. They are a discreet way to take CBD and are suitable for those who prefer a slow-release effect.

Section 3.8.3: Benefits of CBD Edibles

Long-Lasting Effects:

- CBD edibles often provide a longer duration of effects compared to other methods, making them suitable for sustained relief from symptoms.

Precise Dosing:

- Each edible is pre-measured, allowing for precise control over your CBD intake.

Variety:

- CBD edibles come in a wide range of flavors and types, catering to diverse tastes and preferences.

Section 3.8.4: Considerations and Tips

Digestive Processing:

- Keep in mind that the digestive process can affect the onset of effects. Effects may take longer to manifest compared to sublingual methods.

Dosing:

- Start with a low dose, especially if you are new to CBD, and gradually increase it until you find the optimal dose for your needs.

Quality Assurance:

- Choose reputable brands that provide third-party lab testing to ensure product purity and CBD content.

Section 3.8.5: Conclusion

CBD edibles offer a delicious and convenient way to enjoy the potential benefits of CBD. With a wide variety of flavors and dosages, they cater to different preferences and lifestyles. In the following chapters, we will explore additional types of CBD products, their benefits, and considerations for use.

Chapter 3 provides a comprehensive overview of CBD edibles, including their composition, manufacturing processes, dosing, administration methods, benefits, and important considerations for consumers.

CBD Topicals

Section 3.8.6: CBD Topicals

CBD topicals are a unique and popular category of CBD products that are designed for external use. In this section, we will explore the characteristics, benefits, and considerations of CBD topicals in detail.

Section 3.8.7: Introduction to CBD Topicals

What Are CBD Topicals?

- CBD topicals are products infused with CBD extract, typically derived from hemp, that are intended for topical application to the skin. These can include creams, balms, lotions, salves, and more.

Targeted Relief:

CBD topicals are designed to be applied directly to specific areas of the body, making them ideal for targeting localized discomfort, pain, or skin concerns.

Section 3.8.8: How CBD Topicals Are Made

CBD Extract:

- **High-quality CBD extract** is used in the formulation of topicals. This extract is carefully processed to remove impurities while preserving the beneficial compounds.

Formulation:

- CBD extract is combined with other ingredients like carrier oils, essential oils, and sometimes additional active ingredients depending on the specific product's intended use.

Section 3.8.9: Potency and Dosage

Precise Application:

- CBD topicals allow for precise application to the affected area, ensuring that the CBD is concentrated where it's needed most.

Absorption Rate:

- **The absorption rate** of CBD through the skin varies but is generally slower than with other administration methods. Effects may be felt within minutes to hours.

Section 3.9.0: Administration Method

Topical Application:

- CBD topicals are applied directly to the skin, where they are absorbed through the epidermis and can interact with cannabinoid receptors in the skin.

Section 3.9.1: Benefits of CBD Topicals

Localized Relief:

- CBD topicals are excellent for providing targeted relief. They can be used for issues like muscle soreness, joint pain, skin conditions, and more.

No Systemic Effects:

- Unlike orally consumed CBD products, CBD topicals do not enter the bloodstream, so they do not produce systemic effects or affect the entire body.

Moisturizing and Nourishing:

- Many CBD topicals contain ingredients that can moisturize and nourish the skin, leaving it feeling soft and refreshed.

Section 3.9.2: Considerations and Tips

Application:

- Apply CBD topicals generously to the affected area and massage it gently into the skin until it is fully absorbed.

Consistency:

- For the best results, use CBD topicals consistently over time, especially for ongoing skin concerns or discomfort.

Quality Assurance:

- Choose reputable brands that provide third-party lab testing to ensure the purity and CBD content of their products.

Section 3.9.3: Conclusion

CBD topicals offer a unique and effective way to experience the potential benefits of CBD. They are versatile and suitable for addressing a range of localized issues, from muscle soreness to skin conditions. In the following chapters, we will explore additional types of CBD products, their benefits, and considerations for use.

Chapter 3 provides an in-depth exploration of CBD topicals, including their composition, manufacturing processes, dosing, administration methods, benefits, and important considerations for consumers.

CBD Vapes and Inhalables

Section 3.9.4: CBD Vapes and Inhalables

- **CBD vapes and inhalables** offer a rapid and efficient method of consuming cannabidiol. In this section, we will delve into the characteristics, benefits, and considerations associated with these inhalation methods.

Section 3.9.5: Introduction to CBD Vapes and Inhalables

What Are CBD Vapes and Inhalables?

- CBD vapes and inhalables are products designed for inhalation into the lungs. These include vaporizers, vape pens, e-cigarettes, and smokable hemp flower.

Fast-Acting Delivery:

- Inhalation methods provide one of the quickest onset times for CBD effects, making them suitable for those seeking rapid relief.

Section 3.9.5: How CBD Vapes and Inhalables Are Made

CBD Extract:

- **CBD extracts** used for vapes and inhalables must be carefully processed and free of contaminants, as inhaling impurities can pose health risks.

Formulation:

- CBD extract may be combined with other ingredients, such as carrier oils or flavorings, to create vape-ready solutions or e-liquids.

Section 3.9.6: Potency and Dosage

Quick Onset:

- Inhalation methods provide almost instant effects, with users typically feeling the CBD's effects within minutes.

Controlled Dosing:

- Users can control their CBD intake by taking a specific number of puffs or inhaling a measured amount of CBD vapor.

Section 3.9.7: Administration Method

Inhalation:

CBD vapes and inhalables are inhaled directly into the lungs, allowing for rapid absorption into the bloodstream.

Section 3.9.8: Benefits of CBD Vapes and Inhalables

Rapid Relief:

- Inhalation methods offer some of the fastest relief, making them ideal for acute issues like anxiety or pain.

Controlled Dosage:

- Users can easily adjust their CBD intake based on their needs, making it suitable for both beginners and experienced users.

Section 3.9.9: Considerations and Tips

Health and Safety:

- It's essential to choose high-quality products and ensure that the vape pens or devices are clean and well-maintained to minimize health risks associated with vaping.

Dosing Control:

- Start with a low dose and gradually increase it until you achieve the desired effects. This helps prevent overconsumption.

Regulation and Legality:

- Be aware of local regulations regarding vaping and the use of CBD products, as laws can vary by region.

Section 3.9.9.a: Conclusion

CBD vapes and inhalables offer a rapid and efficient means of experiencing the potential benefits of CBD. They are favored for their quick onset and controlled dosing, making them suitable for various users. In the following chapters, we will explore additional types of CBD products, their benefits, and considerations for use.

Chapter 3 provides a comprehensive overview of CBD vapes and inhalables, including their composition, manufacturing processes, dosing, administration methods, benefits, and important considerations for consumers.

Chapter 4: Choosing Quality CBD Products

Reading Labels and Certifications

Section 4.1: Introduction to Quality CBD Products

Selecting high-quality CBD products is crucial for ensuring safety and effectiveness. This chapter will guide you through the process of evaluating CBD products, reading labels, and understanding certifications to make informed choices.

Section 4.2: Understanding CBD Product Labels

CBD Content:

- The label should clearly state the amount of CBD in the product, typically measured in milligrams (mg) per serving or per container.

Full Spectrum, Broad Spectrum, or Isolate:

- Labels should specify whether the product contains full-spectrum CBD (with trace amounts of THC and other cannabinoids), broad-spectrum CBD (without THC but with other cannabinoids), or CBD isolate (pure CBD).

Ingredients List:

- The ingredients list should detail all components used in the product, including any carrier oils, flavorings, or additives.

Serving Size and Dosage:

- The label should provide serving size recommendations and dosage instructions based on the product's potency.

Batch or Lot Number:

- Look for a batch or lot number that can be used to trace the product's manufacturing and testing history.

Expiration Date:

- Check for an expiration date to ensure the product is still safe and effective.

Section 4.3: Third-Party Lab Testing

Importance of Third-Party Testing:

- Reputable CBD manufacturers provide third-party lab testing results to verify the product's potency, purity, and safety.

Certificates of Analysis (COA):

- **COAs** provide detailed information about the product's cannabinoid profile, including CBD and THC content, as well as the absence of harmful contaminants like heavy metals, pesticides, and solvents.

How to Access COAs:

- Look for QR codes, website links, or instructions on the product label that direct you to the product's COA. These should match the batch or lot number on the product.

Section 4.4: Certifications and Quality Standards

USDA Organic Certification:

- **USDA Organic certification** ensures that the hemp used to produce CBD is grown and processed according to strict organic standards, free from synthetic pesticides and fertilizers.

Good Manufacturing Practices (GMP):

- **Products manufactured in GMP**-compliant facilities adhere to quality and safety standards, ensuring consistent and reliable production.

Certified Safety Seals:

- Some CBD products may carry certifications from independent organizations or safety seals, indicating adherence to specific quality and safety standards.

Section 4.5: Choosing the Right CBD Product

Consider Your Needs:

- Determine your specific needs and the type of CBD product that best suits them, whether it's for pain relief, anxiety, sleep, or general wellness.

Start with Reputable Brands:

- Research and choose well-established brands known for transparency, quality, and adherence to industry standards.

Read Customer Reviews:

- **Customer reviews** can provide insights into the product's effectiveness and user experiences.

Consult a Healthcare Professional:

- If you have medical conditions or are taking medications, consult a healthcare provider before using CBD products to ensure they are safe and appropriate for you.

Section 4.6: Conclusion

Choosing quality CBD products is essential for achieving the desired effects while ensuring safety and peace of mind. By carefully reading labels, understanding third-party testing, and considering certifications, you can make informed decisions that align with your wellness goals. In the following chapters, we will explore CBD's potential benefits for specific health concerns and lifestyles.

Chapter 4 provides a comprehensive guide to help you choose high-quality CBD products by understanding product labels, third-party lab testing, and certifications. Making informed choices is vital to ensure that you receive safe and effective CBD products that align with your wellness goals.

Full-Spectrum vs. Broad-Spectrum vs. Isolate

Section 4.7: Introduction to CBD Spectrum Varieties

Selecting the right CBD product involves understanding the spectrum of CBD extracts available in the market. In this chapter, we will delve into the differences between Full-Spectrum, Broad-Spectrum, and Isolate CBD products to help you make informed choices that align with your needs and preferences.

Section 4.8: Full-Spectrum CBD

What Is Full-Spectrum CBD?

- **Full-Spectrum CBD** contains the full range of naturally occurring cannabinoids, terpenes, and other phytochemicals found in the cannabis plant, including THC (but typically in amounts less than 0.3% in compliance with legal regulations).

The Entourage Effect:

- Full-Spectrum CBD is believed to benefit from the **"entourage effect,"** where the combined presence of multiple cannabinoids and terpenes enhances the overall therapeutic effects.

Benefits:

- Full-Spectrum CBD may provide a wide range of potential benefits, including relief from pain, inflammation, anxiety, and sleep disorders.

Section 4.9: Broad-Spectrum CBD

What Is Broad-Spectrum CBD?

- **Broad-Spectrum CBD** also contains a variety of cannabinoids, terpenes, and phytochemicals, but it undergoes an additional refinement process to remove all traces of THC, making it THC-free.

No THC:

- Broad-Spectrum CBD offers the potential benefits of the entourage effect without the presence of THC, making it a suitable choice for individuals who want to avoid THC entirely.

Benefits:

- Broad-Spectrum CBD may provide similar therapeutic benefits as Full-Spectrum CBD without the risk of THC-related effects.

Section 4.1.0: CBD Isolate

What Is CBD Isolate?

- **CBD Isolate** is the purest form of CBD, containing 99% or more pure CBD without any other cannabinoids, terpenes, or phytochemicals.

THC-Free and Flavorless:

- CBD Isolate is entirely THC-free and has no flavor or aroma, making it an ideal choice for those who want to experience the effects of CBD without any other compounds.

Benefits:

- CBD Isolate is favored for its precision in dosing and its suitability for users with sensitivities to THC or other cannabinoids.

Section 4.1.1: Choosing the Right CBD Spectrum

Consider Your Goals:

- To select the right CBD spectrum, consider your wellness goals. Full-Spectrum and Broad-Spectrum CBD may be more appropriate for users seeking the potential benefits of multiple compounds, while CBD Isolate is suitable for those focused solely on CBD.

THC Sensitivity:

- If you are sensitive to THC or live in an area with strict THC regulations, Broad-Spectrum or Isolate CBD may be preferable.

Personal Experience:

- Experimentation may be necessary to determine which spectrum works best for your specific needs and preferences.

Section 4.1.2: Conclusion

Understanding the differences between Full-Spectrum, Broad-Spectrum, and Isolate CBD products is essential for making informed choices. Each spectrum offers distinct advantages, and the right choice depends on your wellness goals, THC sensitivity, and personal experience. In the following chapters, we will explore specific health concerns and lifestyles where each spectrum may be most beneficial.

Chapter 4 provides a comprehensive guide to help you choose the right CBD product spectrum—Full-Spectrum, Broad-Spectrum, or Isolate—based on your wellness goals, THC sensitivity, and personal preferences. Making an informed choice ensures that you receive the CBD product that aligns best with your specific needs.

Understanding Dosage

Section 4.1.3: Introduction to CBD Dosage

Selecting the right CBD product goes hand in hand with understanding how to determine and manage your CBD dosage effectively. In this chapter, we will delve into the intricacies of CBD dosing to help you make informed decisions that align with your needs and wellness goals.

Section 4.1.4: Importance of Proper Dosage

Individual Variation:

- CBD dosage is not one-size-fits-all. It varies from person to person based on factors like body weight, metabolism, and the specific condition being treated.

Maximizing Benefits:

- Proper dosage is crucial for experiencing the potential therapeutic benefits of CBD while minimizing the risk of adverse effects.

Section 4.1.5: Factors Influencing CBD Dosage

Body Weight:

- As a general guideline, individuals with higher body weights may require higher CBD doses to achieve the same effects as those with lower body weights.

Metabolism:

- Faster metabolisms may process CBD more quickly, potentially requiring more frequent dosing.

Severity of Condition:

- The severity of the condition being treated can influence the optimal CBD dosage. More severe conditions may require higher doses.

Tolerance:

- Over time, some individuals may develop a tolerance to CBD, necessitating an adjustment in dosage.

Section 4.1.6: Starting with a Low Dose

The "Start Low and Go Slow" Approach:

- It is advisable to begin with a low CBD dosage, especially if you are new to CBD. This allows you to gauge how your body responds and gradually adjust the dose as needed.

Incremental Increases:

- If you do not experience the desired effects, you can increase your CBD dosage in small increments until you find the optimal dose.

Section 4.1.7: Standard CBD Dosage Recommendations

General Dosage Ranges:

- A common starting dose for adults is 20-40 mg of CBD per day, with the option to increase based on individual response.

Microdosing:

- Some users prefer **microdosing**, which involves taking very small doses of CBD throughout the day, aiming for a cumulative effect.

Consulting a Healthcare Provider:

- *For specific health concerns or if you are taking medications, it's advisable to consult a healthcare provider for personalized dosage recommendations.*

Section 4.1.8: Monitoring and Adjusting Dosage

Keeping a Journal:

- Maintaining a CBD journal to track dosages, effects, and any side effects can be helpful in determining the optimal dosage.

Patience and Persistence:

- Finding the right CBD dosage may require patience and persistence. Be willing to adjust your dosage as needed to achieve the desired results.

Section 4.7: Conclusion

Understanding CBD dosage is a fundamental aspect of selecting quality CBD products that align with your wellness goals. It involves considering individual factors, starting with a low dose, and gradually adjusting until you find the optimal dosage for your needs. In the following chapters, we will explore specific health concerns and lifestyles where CBD dosage plays a critical role in achieving desired outcomes.

Chapter 4 provides an in-depth guide to help you understand CBD dosage, from individual factors influencing dosing to starting with a low dose and gradually adjusting until you find the optimal dosage for your specific needs. Proper dosage is essential for experiencing the potential therapeutic benefits of CBD effectively and safely.

Chapter 5: Benefits of CBD for Physical Health

Pain Management

Section 5.1: Introduction to CBD for Pain Management

CBD has gained recognition for its potential to alleviate various types of pain, making it a promising option for individuals seeking alternative pain management solutions. In this chapter, we will delve into the mechanisms behind CBD's pain-relieving properties and its effectiveness for managing different types of pain.

Section 5.2: Understanding Pain

Types of Pain:

- Pain can be categorized into acute pain (short-term, often caused by injury) and chronic pain (long-lasting, often associated with underlying conditions like arthritis or neuropathy).

The Role of Inflammation:

- **Inflammation** is a common underlying factor in many types of pain, and CBD's anti-inflammatory properties play a crucial role in pain management.

Section 5.3: How CBD Relieves Pain

Interaction with the Endocannabinoid System (ECS):

- CBD interacts with the body's endocannabinoid system, which plays a role in regulating pain perception and inflammation.

Reduction of Inflammation:

- CBD has been shown to reduce inflammation by influencing receptors in the ECS, leading to potential relief from inflammatory pain.

Modulation of Pain Signals:

- CBD can alter pain signals sent to the brain, potentially reducing the perception of pain.

Section 5.4: Effectiveness of CBD for Different Types of Pain

Chronic Pain:

- Studies suggest that CBD may be effective in managing chronic pain conditions such as arthritis, fibromyalgia, and neuropathy.

Muscle and Joint Pain:

- CBD topicals, when applied directly to sore muscles or joints, can offer localized relief.

Migraines and Headaches:

- Some individuals report a reduction in the frequency and severity of migraines and tension headaches with CBD use.

Postoperative Pain:

- CBD may aid in postoperative pain management and recovery.

Section 5.5: Considerations and Precautions

Dosage and Individual Response:

- CBD dosage for pain management varies among individuals, so it's essential to find the right dose for your specific needs through a process of trial and adjustment.

Consulting a Healthcare Provider:

- It's advisable to consult a healthcare provider, particularly if you are considering CBD as an alternative to prescription pain medications or if you have underlying health conditions.

Interactions with Medications:

- CBD may interact with certain medications, so consult your healthcare provider if you are taking prescription drugs.

Section 5.6: Conclusion

CBD offers promising potential for pain management by interacting with the endocannabinoid system, reducing inflammation, and modulating pain signals. Whether you're dealing with chronic pain, muscle soreness, headaches, or postoperative discomfort, CBD may provide a natural and effective alternative or complement to traditional pain management strategies. In the following chapters, we will explore additional aspects of CBD's potential benefits for physical health.

Chapter 5 provides an in-depth exploration of the benefits of CBD for pain management, covering its mechanisms of action, effectiveness for different types of pain, and important considerations for those considering CBD as a pain relief option. CBD's potential to offer natural and effective pain management makes it a valuable addition to the field of healthcare.

Section 5.7: Introduction to CBD for Inflammation Reduction

- Inflammation is a fundamental biological response to injury and infection, but when it becomes chronic, it can contribute to various health problems. CBD, derived from the cannabis plant, has garnered attention for its potential to reduce inflammation naturally. In this chapter, we will explore the mechanisms behind CBD's anti-inflammatory properties and its potential benefits for physical health.

Section 5.8: Understanding Inflammation

Types of Inflammation:

- **Inflammation** can be categorized as acute (short-term and often a response to injury or infection) or chronic (long-lasting and frequently associated with conditions like arthritis, cardiovascular disease, or autoimmune disorders).

The Role of Inflammatory Processes:

- **Chronic inflammation** is recognized as a key factor in the development and progression of various health conditions, making it a focal point in healthcare research.

Section 5.9: How CBD Reduces Inflammation

Interaction with the Endocannabinoid System (ECS):

- CBD interacts with the body's endocannabinoid system, which plays a role in regulating inflammation and immune responses.

Cytokine Modulation:

- CBD may influence the production and release of cytokines, signaling molecules involved in the body's inflammatory response.

Anti-Oxidative Effects:

- CBD's antioxidant properties can help combat oxidative stress, which is closely linked to inflammation.

Section 5.1.0: Conditions Benefiting from CBD's Anti-Inflammatory Properties

Arthritis and Joint Inflammation:

- CBD shows promise in reducing pain and inflammation associated with arthritis and other joint conditions.

Inflammatory Bowel Diseases (IBD):

- Preliminary studies suggest that CBD may alleviate symptoms of conditions like Crohn's disease and ulcerative colitis.

Neuroinflammation:

- CBD's anti-inflammatory effects may have implications for managing neuroinflammatory conditions, including multiple sclerosis.

Skin Conditions:

- Topical CBD products may help soothe skin conditions like eczema and psoriasis by reducing inflammation.

Section 5.1.1: Considerations and Precautions

Dosage and Individual Response:

- CBD dosage for inflammation reduction can vary among individuals, so it's crucial to find the right dose through a process of adjustment.

Consulting a Healthcare Provider:

- If you are considering CBD for managing chronic inflammation related to a specific condition, consult a healthcare provider for guidance.

Interactions with Medications:

- CBD may interact with certain medications, so it's essential to consult with your healthcare provider, especially if you are taking prescription drugs.

Section 5.1.2: Conclusion

CBD's potential to reduce inflammation offers a natural and holistic approach to enhancing physical health and managing conditions associated with chronic inflammation. Whether you're dealing with joint pain, digestive issues, neuroinflammatory conditions, or skin problems, CBD may provide a valuable solution to mitigate inflammation and promote overall well-being. In the following chapters, we will explore additional aspects of CBD's potential benefits for physical health.

Chapter 5 provides an in-depth exploration of the potential benefits of CBD for reducing inflammation. It covers CBD's mechanisms of action, its effectiveness for various conditions involving inflammation, and important considerations for those considering CBD as an anti-inflammatory remedy. CBD's capacity to address inflammation makes it a valuable option in the realm of natural healthcare.

Chapter 5: Benefits of CBD for Physical Health: Neuroprotective Properties

Section 5.1.3: Introduction to CBD's Neuroprotective Properties

The brain is a vital organ, and its health is paramount for overall physical well-being. CBD has gained attention for its potential neuroprotective properties, making it a promising avenue for maintaining and enhancing brain health. In this chapter, we will explore how CBD interacts with the nervous system and its potential benefits in protecting the brain.

Section 5.1.4: Understanding Neuroprotection

Neuroprotection Defined:

- **Neuroprotection** refers to strategies or substances that aim to protect the nervous system, particularly the brain, from damage or degeneration.

Importance of Brain Health:

- **Maintaining brain health** is essential for cognitive function, emotional well-being, and overall quality of life.

Section 5.1.5: How CBD Exerts Neuroprotective Effects

Interaction with the Endocannabinoid System (ECS):

- CBD interacts with the **endocannabinoid system**, which plays a crucial role in regulating various neurological processes, including neuroprotection.

Anti-Inflammatory Effects:

- CBD's **anti-inflammatory** properties may help reduce neuroinflammation, which is often linked to neurodegenerative diseases.

Antioxidant Properties:

- CBD's antioxidative effects can combat oxidative stress, a major contributor to neurological damage.

Neurogenesis Promotion:

- Some studies suggest that CBD may stimulate the growth of new neurons (neurogenesis) in certain brain regions.

Section 5.1.6: Potential Benefits of CBD for Neuroprotection

Neurodegenerative Diseases:

- CBD has shown promise in preclinical and early clinical studies for conditions like Alzheimer's disease, Parkinson's disease, and multiple sclerosis.

Seizure Disorders:

- CBD has gained FDA approval as a treatment for rare seizure disorders like Dravet syndrome and Lennox-Gastaut syndrome.

Stroke Recovery:

- CBD's neuroprotective properties may aid in stroke recovery by reducing the extent of brain damage.

Mood and Anxiety Disorders:

- CBD may offer neuroprotective effects by reducing anxiety and stress, potentially preventing damage related to chronic stress.

Section 5.1.7: Considerations and Precautions

Dosage and Individual Response:

- The optimal CBD dosage for neuroprotection may vary among individuals, so it's important to find the right dose through gradual adjustment.

Consulting a Healthcare Provider:

- If you are considering CBD for neuroprotection, particularly for managing specific neurological conditions, consult a healthcare provider for personalized guidance.

Interactions with Medications:

- CBD may interact with certain medications, so it's crucial to consult with your healthcare provider, especially if you are taking prescription drugs.

Section 5.1.8: Conclusion

CBD's potential neuroprotective properties offer a compelling avenue for maintaining and enhancing brain health. Whether you're concerned about neurodegenerative diseases, seizure disorders, stroke recovery, or mental health, CBD may provide a natural and promising solution to support the well-being of your nervous system. In the following chapters, we will explore additional aspects of CBD's potential benefits for physical health.

Chapter 5 provides an in-depth exploration of the potential neuroprotective benefits of CBD. It covers CBD's mechanisms of action, its effectiveness for various neurological conditions, and important considerations for those considering CBD as a neuroprotective remedy. CBD's capacity to protect and support the nervous system makes it an intriguing option for maintaining brain health.

Chapter 5: Benefits of CBD for Physical Health: Support for Skin Conditions

Section 5.1.9: Introduction to CBD's Support for Skin Conditions

The skin is the body's largest organ and plays a critical role in protecting us from the external environment. Skin conditions can affect not only our appearance but also our physical comfort and overall well-being. CBD has gained recognition for its potential to support various skin conditions. In this chapter, we will explore how CBD interacts with the skin and its potential benefits in managing skin-related issues.

Section 5.2: Common Skin Conditions

Eczema (Atopic Dermatitis):

- **Eczema** is a chronic inflammatory skin condition characterized by red, itchy, and inflamed skin.

Psoriasis:

- **Psoriasis** is an autoimmune condition that leads to the rapid growth of skin cells, resulting in scaling, redness, and discomfort.

Acne:

- **Acne** is a common skin condition caused by clogged pores, leading to pimples, blackheads, and whiteheads.

Aging and Wrinkles:

- As we age, the skin undergoes natural changes, leading to the development of wrinkles and fine lines.

Section 5.2.1: How CBD Supports Skin Health

Interaction with Cannabinoid Receptors in the Skin:

- The skin has its own endocannabinoid system with receptors that interact with CBD. This interaction can influence various skin functions, including inflammation and cell growth.

Anti-Inflammatory Effects:

- CBD's **anti-inflammatory** properties can help reduce skin inflammation, providing relief for conditions like eczema and psoriasis.

Sebum Regulation:

- CBD may regulate sebum production, which is crucial in managing acne by preventing excess oil buildup.

Antioxidant Effects:

- CBD's antioxidant properties can combat oxidative stress and protect the skin from environmental damage.

Section 5.2.2: Potential Benefits of CBD for Skin Conditions

Eczema (Atopic Dermatitis):

- CBD may help reduce inflammation and itching associated with eczema, providing relief for those with this condition.

Psoriasis:

- Some individuals report improved skin comfort and appearance with the use of topical CBD products for psoriasis.

Acne:

- CBD may help reduce acne by controlling sebum production and offering anti-inflammatory effects.

Aging and Wrinkles:

- The antioxidant properties of CBD can potentially slow down the aging process, reducing the appearance of wrinkles and fine lines.

Section 5.2.3: Considerations and Precautions

Topical vs. Oral CBD:

- The choice of application **(topical vs. oral)** depends on the specific skin condition, and it's important to choose the right method for your needs.

Consulting a Dermatologist:

- For severe skin conditions, it's advisable to consult a dermatologist to determine the most appropriate treatment plan, which may include CBD.

Skin Sensitivity:

- Patch testing is recommended, especially if you have sensitive skin, to ensure no adverse reactions to CBD products.

Section 5.2.5: Conclusion

CBD's potential to support skin health and manage various skin conditions offers a natural and holistic approach to improving physical well-being. Whether you're dealing with eczema, psoriasis, acne, or the signs of aging, CBD may provide a valuable solution for nurturing and maintaining healthy, radiant skin. In the following chapters, we will explore additional aspects of CBD's potential benefits for physical health.

Chapter 5 provides an in-depth exploration of the potential benefits of CBD for supporting skin health and managing common skin conditions. It covers CBD's mechanisms of action, its effectiveness for different skin issues, and important considerations for those considering CBD for their skin-related concerns. CBD's capacity to promote healthy skin makes it a compelling option for overall well-being.

Chapter 5: Benefits of CBD for Physical Health: Cardiovascular Health

Section 5.2.6: Introduction to CBD's Impact on Cardiovascular Health

A healthy cardiovascular system is fundamental to overall physical well-being. CBD has gained attention for its potential to positively affect cardiovascular health. In this chapter, we will explore the connection between CBD and the cardiovascular system, as well as its potential benefits in promoting heart health.

Section 5.2.7: Understanding Cardiovascular Health

The Cardiovascular System:

- **The cardiovascular system** consists of the heart, blood vessels, and blood, and is responsible for pumping oxygen and nutrients throughout the body.

Cardiovascular Conditions:

- **Cardiovascular health** issues include hypertension (high blood pressure), atherosclerosis (hardening of the arteries), and heart disease.

Section 5.2.8: How CBD May Impact Cardiovascular Health

Blood Pressure Regulation:

- Some studies suggest that CBD may help regulate blood pressure, potentially reducing hypertension.

Anti-Inflammatory Effects:

- **CBD's anti-inflammatory** properties can benefit the cardiovascular system by reducing inflammation within blood vessels.

Stress and Anxiety Reduction:

- CBD may help reduce stress and anxiety, which can contribute to heart health by lowering the risk of high blood pressure and heart disease.

Antioxidant Properties:

- CBD's **antioxidant** effects can protect the heart and blood vessels from oxidative stress and damage.

Section 5.2.9: Potential Benefits of CBD for Cardiovascular Health

Blood Pressure Management:

- CBD may help manage **blood pressure,** reducing the risk of hypertension and its associated complications.

Atherosclerosis Prevention:

- By reducing inflammation and oxidative stress, CBD may help prevent the development of atherosclerosis.

Heart Disease Management:

- While more research is needed, CBD shows potential for managing certain aspects of heart disease.

Stress and Anxiety Reduction:

- CBD's ability to reduce stress and anxiety may contribute to a healthier cardiovascular system.

Section 5.3: Considerations and Precautions

Dosage and Individual Response:

- The appropriate CBD dosage for cardiovascular health may vary among individuals, so it's crucial to find the right dose through gradual adjustment.

Consulting a Healthcare Provider:

- If you have existing cardiovascular conditions or are taking heart-related medications, consult a healthcare provider for personalized guidance on using CBD.

Medication Interactions:

- CBD may interact with certain medications, so it's important to consult with your healthcare provider, especially if you are taking prescription drugs for heart health.

Section 5.3.1: Conclusion

CBD's potential to positively impact cardiovascular health offers a holistic approach to maintaining a healthy heart and blood vessels. Whether you're concerned about high blood pressure, atherosclerosis, heart disease, or stress-related factors that affect the heart, CBD may provide a valuable tool for promoting cardiovascular wellness. In the following chapters, we will explore additional aspects of CBD's potential benefits for physical health.

Chapter 5 provides an in-depth exploration of the potential benefits of CBD for cardiovascular health. It covers CBD's mechanisms of action, its effectiveness in promoting heart health, and important considerations for those considering CBD **for** cardiovascular wellness. CBD's capacity to support cardiovascular health makes it a compelling option for overall well-being.

Chapter 5: Benefits of CBD for Physical Health: Digestive Health

Section 5.3.2: Introduction to CBD's Impact on Digestive Health

A healthy digestive system is essential for overall physical well-being. CBD has gained attention for its potential to positively affect digestive health. In this chapter, we will explore the connection between CBD and the digestive system, as well as its potential benefits in promoting a well-functioning gut.

Section 5.3.3: Understanding Digestive Health

The Digestive System:

- The **digestive system** processes food, extracts nutrients, and eliminates waste. A well-functioning gut is critical for nutrient absorption and overall health.

Digestive Disorders:

- Digestive health issues include conditions like irritable bowel syndrome (IBS), inflammatory bowel disease (IBD), and acid reflux.

Section 5.3.4: How CBD May Impact Digestive Health

Anti-Inflammatory Effects:

- CBD's **anti-inflammatory** properties can help reduce inflammation in the digestive tract, potentially alleviating symptoms of conditions like IBS and IBD.

Pain and Discomfort Reduction:

- CBD may help reduce abdominal pain and discomfort associated with digestive conditions.

Nausea and Vomiting Control:

- Some studies suggest that CBD can help manage **nausea and vomiting,** making it beneficial for individuals undergoing chemotherapy or dealing with chronic nausea.

Stress Reduction:

- **Stress** can exacerbate digestive issues, and CBD's ability to reduce stress and anxiety may have a positive impact on gut health.

Section 5.3.5: Potential Benefits of CBD for Digestive Health

Irritable Bowel Syndrome (IBS):

- CBD may help manage **IBS** symptoms, including abdominal pain, bloating, and altered bowel habits.

Inflammatory Bowel Disease (IBD):

- While more research is needed, CBD shows potential in reducing inflammation and improving the quality of life for individuals with IBD.

Nausea and Vomiting:

- CBD may be a useful tool for managing **nausea and vomiting**, particularly for individuals undergoing cancer treatments.

Gastroesophageal Reflux Disease (GERD):

- Some individuals find relief from acid reflux symptoms with the use of CBD.

Section 5.3.6: Considerations and Precautions

Dosage and Individual Response:

- The appropriate CBD dosage for digestive health may vary among individuals, so it's crucial to find the right dose through gradual adjustment.

Consulting a Healthcare Provider:

- If you have existing digestive conditions or are taking medications for digestive health, **consult a healthcare provider** for personalized guidance on using CBD.

Medication Interactions:

- CBD may interact with certain **medications**, so it's important to consult with your healthcare provider, especially if you are taking prescription drugs for digestive issues.

Section 5.6: Conclusion

CBD's potential to promote digestive health offers a holistic approach to maintaining a well-functioning gut and managing various digestive conditions. Whether you're concerned about IBS, IBD, nausea, or acid reflux, CBD may provide a valuable tool for supporting digestive wellness. In the following chapters, we will explore additional aspects of CBD's potential benefits for physical health.

Chapter 5 provides an in-depth exploration of the potential benefits of CBD for digestive health. It covers CBD's mechanisms of action, its effectiveness in promoting gut health, and important considerations for those considering CBD for digestive wellness. CBD's capacity to support digestive health makes it a compelling option for overall well-being.

Chapter 6: Benefits of CBD for Mental Health: Depression and Mood Disorders

Section 6.1: Introduction to CBD's Impact on Depression and Mood Disorders

Depression and mood disorders can profoundly affect an individual's mental health and overall well-being. CBD has garnered attention for its potential to alleviate symptoms of depression and improve mood. In this chapter, we will explore the connection between CBD and mental health, with a specific focus on its effectiveness in managing depression and mood disorders.

Section 6.2: Understanding Depression and Mood Disorders

Depression Defined:

- Mood disorders encompass a wide range of conditions, including bipolar disorder, major depressive disorder, and seasonal affective disorder.

Section 6.3: How CBD May Impact Depression and Mood Disorders

Neurotransmitter Regulation:

- CBD may influence the balance of various neurotransmitters, including serotonin, which plays a crucial role in mood regulation.

Hippocampal Neurogenesis:

- Some studies suggest that CBD may stimulate the growth of new neurons in the hippocampus, a region of the brain associated with mood and memory.

Anti-Anxiety Effects:

- CBD's ability to reduce anxiety can be particularly beneficial for individuals with comorbid anxiety and depression.

Section 6.4: Potential Benefits of CBD for Depression and Mood Disorders

Major Depressive Disorder (MDD):

- CBD may help alleviate symptoms of MDD, such as persistent sadness and loss of interest.

Bipolar Disorder:

- While more research is needed, CBD shows promise in mood stabilization for individuals with bipolar disorder.

Seasonal Affective Disorder (SAD):

- CBD may offer relief for individuals with SAD, especially during the winter months when symptoms typically worsen.

Comorbid Anxiety and Depression:

- CBD's potential to alleviate both anxiety and depression can benefit individuals with comorbid conditions.

Section 6.5: Considerations and Precautions

Dosage and Individual Response:

- Finding the right CBD dosage for depression and mood disorders may require individual adjustment.

Consulting a Mental Health Professional:

- If you have been diagnosed with a mood disorder or severe depression, it is advisable to consult a mental health professional to discuss the incorporation of CBD into your treatment plan.

Medication Interactions:

- CBD may interact with certain medications, so it's important to consult with your healthcare provider, especially if you are taking prescription drugs for mood disorders.

Section 6.6: Conclusion

CBD's potential to alleviate symptoms of depression and mood disorders offers a natural and holistic approach to promoting mental well-being. Whether you're dealing with major depressive disorder, bipolar disorder, seasonal affective disorder, or comorbid anxiety and depression, CBD may provide a valuable tool for managing these conditions and enhancing overall mental health. In the following chapters, we will explore additional aspects of CBD's potential benefits for mental health.

Chapter 6 provides an exhaustive exploration of the potential benefits of CBD for managing depression and mood disorders. It covers CBD's mechanisms of action, its effectiveness in addressing different mood disorders, and important considerations for those considering CBD for their mental well-being. CBD's capacity to support mental health makes it a compelling option for overall psychological and emotional well-being.

Chapter 7: CBD for Specific Conditions

Introduction to CBD's Application for Specific Health Conditions

CBD has shown promise in alleviating symptoms and improving quality of life for individuals with various health conditions. In this chapter, we will explore the specific applications of CBD for a range of health issues, including chronic pain, epilepsy, insomnia, and more. By examining the latest research and real-world experiences, we aim to provide comprehensive insights into how CBD can be used to address specific health concerns.

Section 7.1: CBD for Epilepsy and Seizures

Epilepsy and Seizures Defined:

- Epilepsy is a neurological disorder characterized by recurrent seizures, which can vary in severity and frequency. Seizures result from abnormal electrical activity in the brain.

CBD's Antiepileptic Effects:

- CBD has gained attention for its potential to reduce seizure frequency and severity in individuals with treatment-resistant epilepsy.

Research and Evidence:

- Clinical trials have demonstrated the efficacy of CBD in reducing seizures, leading to FDA approval of CBD-based medications for certain forms of epilepsy, such as Dravet syndrome and Lennox-Gastaut syndrome.

Real-World Impact:

- Many individuals with epilepsy have reported significant improvements in seizure control and quality of life after incorporating CBD into their treatment regimens.

Section 7.2: CBD for Chronic Pain Conditions

Chronic Pain Defined:

- Chronic pain refers to persistent pain lasting for weeks, months, or even years, often resulting from conditions like arthritis, fibromyalgia, or injury.

CBD's Mechanisms in Pain Management:

- CBD interacts with receptors in the endocannabinoid system, modulating pain perception and reducing inflammation, making it a promising option for chronic pain management.

Research and Evidence:

- Numerous studies have demonstrated CBD's effectiveness in reducing chronic pain, with some individuals experiencing significant relief without the adverse side effects associated with traditional pain medications.

Real-World Applications:

- Patients with conditions like arthritis, fibromyalgia, neuropathy, and multiple sclerosis have reported improvements in pain levels and overall quality of life with the use of CBD products.

Section 7.3: CBD for Arthritis and Joint Health

Arthritis Defined:

- Arthritis is a common condition characterized by inflammation and stiffness in the joints, leading to pain and reduced mobility.

CBD's Anti-Inflammatory Effects:

- CBD's anti-inflammatory properties may help alleviate symptoms of arthritis by reducing joint inflammation and associated pain.

Research and Evidence:

- Some studies have shown promising results regarding the use of CBD for arthritis pain relief, although more research is needed to fully understand its efficacy and optimal dosage.

Real-World Impact:

- Many individuals with arthritis have reported reduced pain and improved joint function after incorporating CBD into their treatment regimens, either topically or orally.

Section 7.4: CBD for Multiple Sclerosis (MS)

Multiple Sclerosis Defined:

- Multiple sclerosis is a chronic autoimmune disease that affects the central nervous system, leading to symptoms such as muscle spasms, pain, and impaired mobility.

CBD's Neuroprotective Effects:

- CBD's potential to protect neurons and reduce inflammation may offer benefits for individuals with MS by alleviating symptoms and slowing disease progression.

Research and Evidence:

- While research on CBD specifically for MS is limited, some studies suggest that CBD may help manage symptoms such as muscle spasms and pain in individuals with MS.

Real-World Impact:

- Patients with MS have reported improvements in symptoms such as spasticity, pain, and sleep disturbances with the use of CBD products, contributing to enhanced quality of life.

Section 7.5: CBD for Cancer Support

Cancer Support Defined:

- CBD may offer supportive care for individuals undergoing cancer treatment, addressing symptoms such as pain, nausea, and loss of appetite.

Palliative Care and Symptom Management:

- CBD's analgesic, antiemetic, and appetite-stimulating properties can provide relief for cancer patients experiencing pain, chemotherapy-induced nausea, and appetite loss.

Research and Evidence:

- While more research is needed, preliminary studies and anecdotal evidence suggest that CBD may complement traditional cancer treatments by improving symptom management and quality of life.

Real-World Impact:

- Many cancer patients have reported relief from treatment-related symptoms and improved well-being with the use of CBD products as part of their comprehensive care plans.

Section 7.6: CBD for Inflammatory Bowel Disease (IBD)

Inflammatory Bowel Disease Defined:

- Inflammatory bowel disease (IBD) encompasses conditions such as Crohn's disease and ulcerative colitis, characterized by chronic inflammation of the digestive tract.

CBD's Anti-Inflammatory Effects:

- CBD's ability to reduce inflammation may benefit individuals with IBD by alleviating symptoms such as abdominal pain, diarrhea, and inflammation.

Research and Evidence:

- While research on CBD for IBD is still in its early stages, some studies suggest that CBD may help manage symptoms and improve quality of life for individuals with these conditions.

Real-World Impact:

- Patients with IBD have reported reductions in symptoms such as pain, diarrhea, and fatigue with the use of CBD products, contributing to better disease management and overall well-being.

Section 7.7: Conclusion

CBD shows significant promise as a therapeutic agent for addressing a diverse array of health conditions, ranging from epilepsy and chronic pain to arthritis, multiple sclerosis, cancer support, and inflammatory bowel disease. By understanding the mechanisms of action, accumulating research evidence, and real-world experiences, individuals and healthcare professionals can make informed decisions about incorporating CBD into treatment regimens for specific health concerns.

Chapter 7 provides an in-depth exploration of the specific applications of CBD for various health conditions. It covers the mechanisms of action, research evidence, and real-world experiences associated with using CBD to address epilepsy, chronic pain, arthritis, multiple sclerosis, cancer support, and inflammatory bowel disease.

Chapter 8: CBD for Pets

Section 8.1: Introduction to CBD for Pets

- CBD's popularity isn't limited to humans; pet owners are increasingly turning to CBD to address various health concerns in their furry companions. In this chapter, we will explore the benefits, dosage considerations, safety, and real-life stories of CBD for pets, including dogs and cats.

Section 8.2: Benefits for Dogs and Cats

Anxiety and Stress Relief:

- CBD may help alleviate anxiety and stress in pets, particularly during thunderstorms, fireworks, separation anxiety, or visits to the veterinarian.

Pain Management:

- CBD's anti-inflammatory and analgesic properties make it beneficial for managing pain in pets, whether due to arthritis, injury, or post-surgery recovery.

Seizure Control:

- Similar to humans, CBD may help reduce the frequency and severity of seizures in dogs and cats with epilepsy or other seizure disorders.

Skin Conditions:

- CBD's anti-inflammatory and antibacterial properties can aid in the management of skin conditions like allergies, hot spots, and dermatitis in pets.

Digestive Health:

- CBD may help regulate digestion, alleviate nausea, and reduce inflammation in the gastrointestinal tract, making it beneficial for pets with digestive issues.

Section 8.3: Dosage and Safety

Dosage Guidelines:

- Determining the appropriate CBD dosage for pets depends on factors such as weight, age, health condition, and individual response. It's crucial to start with a low dose and gradually increase as needed while monitoring for any adverse effects.

Pet-Specific CBD Products:

- Pet CBD products come in various forms, including oils, treats, capsules, and topicals, each with its own recommended dosage and administration method. It's essential to choose products specifically formulated for pets to ensure safety and effectiveness.

Consultation with Veterinarian:

- Before starting your pet on a CBD regimen, consult with a veterinarian familiar with CBD use in animals. They can provide personalized guidance based on your pet's health status and potential interactions with other medications.

Quality and Safety Considerations:

- Opt for high-quality CBD products sourced from reputable manufacturers that undergo third-party testing for potency and purity. Look for products made from organic hemp extract and free from harmful additives or contaminants.

Section 8.4: Real-Life Stories of CBD for Pets

Case Studies:

- Real-life stories of pet owners who have used CBD for their furry companions can provide valuable insights into its effectiveness and impact on their pets' well-being.

Testimonials:

- Pet owners often share testimonials about the positive effects of CBD on their pets, including improvements in mobility, behavior, and overall quality of life.

Success Stories:

- From senior dogs finding relief from arthritis pain to anxious cats experiencing calmness and relaxation, there are numerous success stories highlighting the benefits of CBD for pets across various health conditions.

Section 8.5: Conclusion

CBD offers promising potential as a natural remedy for addressing a wide range of health issues in dogs and cats. By understanding the benefits, dosage considerations, safety precautions, and real-life stories of CBD for pets, pet owners can make informed decisions about incorporating CBD into their pets' wellness routines. As research continues to evolve, CBD may continue to emerge as a valuable tool for supporting the health and well-being of our beloved furry companions.

Chapter 8 provides an in-depth exploration of the benefits, dosage considerations, safety precautions, and real-life stories of CBD for pets, offering pet owners valuable insights into incorporating CBD into their pets' wellness routines.

Chapter 9: Potential Side Effects and Risks

Section 9.1: Introduction to Potential Side Effects and Risks

While CBD offers various potential benefits, it's essential to understand that like any supplement or medication, it may also carry certain risks and side effects. In this chapter, we will explore the common side effects, drug interactions, and safety concerns associated with CBD use.

Section 9.2: Common Side Effects

Dry Mouth (Xerostomia):

- Dry mouth is a common side effect reported by individuals using CBD, often resulting from decreased saliva production. This may lead to feelings of thirst and discomfort.

Drowsiness and Fatigue:

- Some individuals may experience drowsiness or fatigue after taking CBD, especially at higher doses. This side effect is more common with certain formulations or when CBD is combined with other sedating substances.

Changes in Appetite:

- CBD may influence appetite in some individuals, leading to increased or decreased hunger. While this effect is generally mild, it may impact dietary habits and weight management.

Gastrointestinal Disturbances:

- CBD use can sometimes cause gastrointestinal symptoms such as nausea, diarrhea, or stomach discomfort. These effects are typically mild and transient but may occur in sensitive individuals.

Section 9.3: Drug Interactions

Cytochrome P450 Enzyme Interaction:

- CBD interacts with the cytochrome P450 enzyme system in the liver, which plays a crucial role in metabolizing many medications. As a result, CBD may affect the metabolism of certain drugs, leading to altered blood levels and potential adverse effects.

Potential Interactions with Medications:

- CBD may interact with medications that are metabolized by the cytochrome P450 system, including blood thinners, antiepileptic drugs, antidepressants, and certain antipsychotics. This can increase the risk of side effects or reduce the effectiveness of these medications.

Consultation with Healthcare Provider:

- It's essential to consult with a healthcare provider before using CBD, especially if you are taking prescription medications. They can assess your individual risk profile and provide guidance on potential interactions and dosage adjustments.

Section 9.4: Safety Concerns

Quality and Purity:

- Ensuring the quality and purity of CBD products is essential for safety. Poorly regulated products may contain contaminants or inconsistent levels of CBD, posing risks to consumers.

THC Content:

- Some CBD products may contain trace amounts of THC, the psychoactive compound found in cannabis. While these levels are typically low and not intoxicating, they may still pose risks, especially for individuals sensitive to THC or subject to drug testing.

Pregnancy and Lactation:

- Limited research exists on the safety of CBD use during pregnancy and lactation. Due to potential risks to the developing fetus or breastfeeding infant, it's advisable to avoid CBD use in these populations unless under the guidance of a healthcare provider.

Adverse Reactions:

- While rare, some individuals may experience allergic reactions or sensitivity to CBD or other ingredients in CBD products. It's essential to discontinue use and seek medical attention if you experience severe or concerning symptoms.

Section 9.5: Conclusion

While CBD offers promising potential for various health benefits, it's essential to be aware of the potential side effects, drug interactions, and safety concerns associated with its use. By understanding these risks and taking appropriate precautions, individuals can make informed decisions about incorporating CBD into their wellness routines while minimizing potential harm.

Chapter 9 provides an in-depth exploration of the potential side effects and risks associated with CBD use, including common side effects, drug interactions, and safety concerns. By understanding these factors, individuals can make informed decisions about CBD use and mitigate potential risks while maximizing potential benefits.

Chapter 10: CBD Research and Future Potential

Section 10.1: Introduction to CBD Research

Research into the therapeutic potential of CBD is rapidly expanding, driven by growing interest from scientists, healthcare professionals, and the public alike. In this chapter, we will explore the current state of CBD research, emerging areas of study, and the regulatory challenges that shape the future of CBD's potential.

Section 10.2: Ongoing Research

Clinical Trials:

- Numerous clinical trials are underway to investigate the efficacy and safety of CBD for various health conditions, including epilepsy, chronic pain, anxiety, and more. These studies aim to provide robust scientific evidence to support CBD's therapeutic use.

Mechanisms of Action:

- Research continues to elucidate the mechanisms by which CBD exerts its effects on the body, including its interactions with the endocannabinoid system, neurotransmitter systems, and inflammatory pathways. Understanding these mechanisms is crucial for optimizing CBD-based treatments.

Long-Term Effects:

- Long-term studies are needed to assess the safety and efficacy of prolonged CBD use, particularly in vulnerable populations such as children, elderly individuals, and those with chronic health conditions. These studies will help identify any potential risks associated with extended CBD use.

Section 10.3: Emerging Areas of Study

Neurological Disorders:

- CBD shows promise in the treatment of various neurological disorders, including Alzheimer's disease, Parkinson's disease, and Huntington's disease. Research in this area aims to elucidate CBD's neuroprotective and neuroregenerative properties.

Psychiatric Conditions:

- Studies are exploring the potential of CBD in managing psychiatric conditions such as schizophrenia, bipolar disorder, and post-traumatic stress disorder (PTSD). CBD's anxiolytic and mood-stabilizing effects make it a promising candidate for adjunctive therapy in mental health care.

Cancer Treatment:

- Research suggests that CBD may complement traditional cancer treatments by enhancing chemotherapy efficacy, reducing chemotherapy-induced side effects, and inhibiting tumor growth. Clinical trials are investigating CBD's role in cancer therapy and supportive care.

Metabolic Disorders:

- Preliminary research indicates that CBD may have metabolic effects, including regulating appetite, metabolism, and insulin sensitivity. Studies in this area aim to explore CBD's potential in managing obesity, diabetes, and metabolic syndrome.

Section 10.4: Regulatory Challenges

Legal Status:

- The legal status of CBD varies widely across countries and regions, posing challenges for researchers, healthcare professionals, and consumers. Regulatory frameworks continue to evolve, impacting CBD research, production, and access.

Quality Control:

- Ensuring the quality and consistency of CBD products is essential for conducting reliable research and ensuring consumer safety. Regulatory agencies face challenges in establishing and enforcing quality control standards for the rapidly growing CBD industry.

Access to Research Funding:

- Despite increasing interest in CBD research, securing funding for studies can be challenging due to regulatory restrictions, stigma associated with cannabis, and competition for research funding in other areas of medicine. Increased investment in CBD research is needed to support further scientific exploration.

Section 10.5: Conclusion

CBD research holds immense promise for advancing our understanding of its therapeutic potential and improving health outcomes for individuals worldwide. By addressing ongoing research gaps, exploring emerging areas of study, and navigating regulatory challenges, we can unlock the full potential of CBD as a safe and effective treatment option for a wide range of health conditions.

Chapter 10 provides an in-depth exploration of CBD research and future potential, covering ongoing studies, emerging areas of study, and regulatory challenges. By addressing these research gaps and overcoming regulatory hurdles, we can harness the full therapeutic potential of CBD and improve health outcomes for individuals globally.

Chapter 11: How to Incorporate CBD into Your Wellness Routine

Section 11.1: Introduction to CBD Integration

CBD has gained popularity as a natural remedy for various health concerns, but incorporating it into your wellness routine requires careful consideration and planning. In this chapter, we will explore the steps to effectively integrate CBD into your daily regimen, including consulting with healthcare professionals, finding the right dosage, and creating a personalized CBD wellness plan.

Section 11.2: Consulting with Healthcare Professionals

Assessment of Health Goals:

- Begin by discussing your health goals and concerns with a healthcare professional, such as a doctor or pharmacist. They can help assess whether CBD is suitable for your specific needs and provide personalized recommendations.

Review of Medical History:

- Provide your healthcare provider with a comprehensive medical history, including any pre-existing health conditions, medications, supplements, or allergies. This information will help guide their assessment of CBD's suitability and safety for you.

Guidance on CBD Use:

- Healthcare professionals can offer valuable guidance on incorporating CBD into your wellness routine, including dosage recommendations, potential interactions with medications, and monitoring for side effects or adverse reactions.

Section 11.3: Finding the Right Dosage

Start Low and Go Slow:

- When starting with CBD, it's essential to begin with a low dosage and gradually increase it over time as needed. This allows you to assess your individual response and minimize the risk of adverse effects.

Titration Process:

- Experiment with different dosages to find the optimal level that provides the desired benefits without causing unwanted side effects. Keep a journal to track your CBD usage, dosage, and any changes in symptoms or well-being.

Consider Individual Factors:

- Dosage requirements can vary significantly among individuals based on factors such as body weight, metabolism, health condition, and sensitivity to CBD. What works for one person may not necessarily work for another.

Section 11.4: Creating a CBD Wellness Plan

Identify Wellness Goals:

- Define clear wellness goals you hope to achieve with CBD, whether it's managing chronic pain, reducing anxiety, improving sleep quality, or enhancing overall well-being.

Select Suitable CBD Products:

- Choose CBD products that align with your wellness goals and preferences, such as oils, capsules, edibles, topicals, or vape products. Consider factors like bioavailability, onset time, and convenience of administration.

Establish a Routine:

- Incorporate CBD into your daily routine by establishing a consistent dosing schedule and administration method. This helps maintain steady blood levels of CBD and enhances its effectiveness over time.

Monitor Progress and Adjust as Needed:

- Regularly assess your progress towards achieving your wellness goals and adjust your CBD dosage or product selection as necessary. Be patient and persistent, as it may take time to experience the full benefits of CBD.

Section 11.5: Conclusion

Incorporating CBD into your wellness routine requires thoughtful consideration, collaboration with healthcare professionals, and a personalized approach tailored to your individual needs and goals. By following these steps and staying informed, you can maximize the potential benefits of CBD and enhance your overall health and well-being.

Chapter 11 provides a comprehensive guide to integrating CBD into your wellness routine, covering key steps such as consulting with healthcare professionals, finding the right dosage, and creating a personalized CBD wellness plan. By following these recommendations and staying proactive in managing your CBD usage, you can optimize its effectiveness and achieve your wellness goals.

Chapter 12: The Future of CBD

Section 12.1: Introduction to Future Trends and Innovations

The landscape of CBD is constantly evolving, driven by ongoing research, technological advancements, and shifting regulatory frameworks. In this chapter, we will explore the future trends and innovations shaping the trajectory of CBD, its place in modern healthcare, and its global perspective.

Section 12.2: Trends and Innovations

Nanoencapsulation Technology:

- Advancements in nanoencapsulation technology enable the creation of water-soluble CBD formulations with enhanced bioavailability and rapid onset of action. These innovations are revolutionizing the way CBD is consumed and absorbed by the body.

Microdosing:

- The practice of microdosing involves taking small, subtherapeutic doses of CBD regularly throughout the day. This approach aims to maintain steady blood levels of CBD, optimizing its therapeutic effects while minimizing the risk of side effects.

Targeted Delivery Systems:

- Targeted delivery systems, such as transdermal patches, nasal sprays, and intraoral formulations, allow for precise dosing and localized administration of CBD to specific areas of the body. These delivery methods offer enhanced efficacy and convenience for users.

Personalized Medicine:

- The future of CBD lies in personalized medicine, where treatment regimens are tailored to individual needs, preferences, and genetic factors. Advances in pharmacogenomics and predictive analytics will enable healthcare providers to optimize CBD therapy for each patient.

Section 12.3: CBD's Place in Modern Healthcare

Integration into Clinical Practice:

- As the body of evidence supporting CBD's therapeutic potential continues to grow, healthcare providers are increasingly integrating CBD into their clinical practice. CBD is being used as adjunctive therapy for various health conditions, including chronic pain, anxiety, epilepsy, and more.

Holistic Approach to Wellness:

- CBD's holistic approach to wellness aligns with the shift towards personalized, preventive healthcare. It complements conventional treatments by addressing the root causes of health imbalances and promoting overall well-being.

Patient Empowerment:

- CBD empowers patients to take control of their health and explore natural, alternative treatment options. By providing access to safe, effective CBD products and educational resources, individuals can make informed decisions about their wellness journey.

Section 12.4: Global Perspective on CBD

Diverse Regulatory Landscapes:

- The regulatory landscape for CBD varies significantly from country to country, ranging from strict prohibition to legalization for medical or recreational use. Harmonizing regulations and establishing international standards will facilitate global access to high-quality CBD products.

Cultural Acceptance and Stigma:

- Cultural attitudes towards cannabis and CBD influence its acceptance and usage patterns worldwide. Education and awareness campaigns are essential for dispelling myths, reducing stigma, and fostering informed discussions about CBD's potential benefits and risks.

International Research Collaboration:

- Collaboration among researchers, healthcare professionals, and policymakers on a global scale is crucial for advancing CBD research, sharing best practices, and shaping evidence-based policies. Multidisciplinary efforts will drive innovation and drive the growth of the CBD industry.

Section 12.5: Conclusion

The future of CBD is characterized by innovation, integration into modern healthcare, and a global perspective that transcends borders. By embracing emerging trends and technologies, leveraging CBD's potential in clinical practice, and fostering international collaboration, we can unlock the full promise of CBD as a safe, effective, and accessible tool for promoting health and well-being worldwide.

Chapter 12 provides an extensive exploration of the future of CBD, covering emerging trends and innovations, its evolving role in modern healthcare, and its global perspective. By understanding these dynamics and embracing opportunities for growth and collaboration, we can shape a future where CBD contributes to healthier, more empowered communities around the globe.

Chapter 13: Frequently Asked Questions about CBD

Section 13.1: Addressing Common Queries

Q1: What is CBD, and how does it differ from THC?

- CBD, or cannabidiol, is a natural compound found in cannabis plants. Unlike THC (tetrahydrocannabinol), CBD is non-intoxicating and does not produce the "high" typically associated with cannabis use. Instead, it is known for its potential therapeutic effects on various health conditions.

Q2: Is CBD legal?

- The legal status of CBD varies depending on factors such as its source (hemp-derived vs. marijuana-derived), the concentration of THC, and local regulations. In many regions, hemp-derived CBD with less than 0.3% THC is legal for sale and consumption, but it's essential to check local laws and regulations.

Q3: How does CBD work in the body?

- CBD interacts with the endocannabinoid system (ECS), a complex network of receptors and neurotransmitters involved in regulating various physiological processes such as mood, pain sensation, appetite, and immune function. By modulating ECS activity, CBD may exert its therapeutic effects.

Q4: What are the potential health benefits of CBD?

- CBD has been studied for its potential benefits in managing a wide range of health conditions, including chronic pain, anxiety, depression, epilepsy, inflammation, insomnia, and more. While research is ongoing, many individuals report positive effects from using CBD for various wellness purposes.

Q5: How do I choose a high-quality CBD product?

- When selecting a CBD product, it's essential to consider factors such as the source of the hemp, extraction method, third-party testing for potency and purity, and product transparency (e.g., clear labeling, certificates of analysis). Opt for reputable brands with a track record of quality and transparency.

Section 13.2: Clarifying Misconceptions

Q6: Will CBD get me high?

- No, CBD is non-intoxicating and does not produce psychoactive effects. Unlike THC, which binds directly to cannabinoid receptors in the brain, CBD interacts with receptors indirectly and does not induce the euphoric "high" associated with cannabis use.

Q7: Is CBD addictive?

- There is no evidence to suggest that CBD is addictive or habit-forming. In fact, CBD has been studied for its potential role in managing addiction and withdrawal symptoms associated with substance abuse.

Q8: Can I overdose on CBD?

- CBD is generally well-tolerated, even at high doses, and there is no known risk of overdose. However, taking excessively high doses may increase the risk of side effects such as drowsiness, dry mouth, or gastrointestinal discomfort.

Q9: Will CBD show up on a drug test?

- While pure CBD itself is unlikely to trigger a positive result on standard drug tests, some CBD products may contain trace amounts of THC, which could potentially result in a positive test result, especially with frequent or high-dose use. It's essential to choose THC-free products or be mindful of THC content if drug testing is a concern.

Q10: Can I give CBD to my pet?

- Yes, CBD products formulated specifically for pets are available and may offer benefits for managing various health conditions in dogs, cats, and other animals. However, it's crucial to consult with a veterinarian before giving CBD to pets to ensure safety and appropriate dosing.

Section 13.3: Conclusion

By addressing common questions and misconceptions about CBD, individuals can make informed decisions about its use and navigate the rapidly evolving landscape of CBD products and regulations. Education and awareness play a crucial role in promoting responsible CBD consumption and maximizing its potential benefits for health and wellness.

Chapter 13 provides a comprehensive overview of frequently asked questions about CBD, addressing common queries and clarifying misconceptions to empower individuals with accurate information and guidance for incorporating CBD into their wellness routines.

Chapter 14: Success Stories and Testimonials

Section 14.1: Introduction to Real-Life Accounts

CBD has touched the lives of countless individuals around the world, offering hope and relief for a wide range of health conditions. In this chapter, we will explore real-life success stories and testimonials from individuals who have experienced the transformative effects of CBD.

Section 14.2: Chronic Pain Relief

Sarah's Story (United States):

Sarah, a 45-year-old woman from California, struggled with chronic back pain for years due to a spinal injury. After trying various treatments with limited success, she turned to CBD as a last resort. Within weeks of starting a CBD oil regimen, Sarah noticed a significant reduction in pain and stiffness, allowing her to regain mobility and improve her quality of life.

Section 14.3: Anxiety and Stress Management

David's Story (United Kingdom):

David, a 30-year-old professional from London, battled with anxiety and panic attacks for most of his adult life. Prescription medications provided temporary relief but came with undesirable side effects. Upon discovering CBD, David found a natural alternative that helped him manage his symptoms effectively. With regular use of CBD capsules, David experienced a newfound sense of calmness and mental clarity, enabling him to navigate daily challenges with greater ease.

Section 14.4: Epilepsy Control

Emma's Story (Australia):

Emma, a 10-year-old girl from Sydney, was diagnosed with Dravet syndrome, a severe form of epilepsy, at a young age. Despite trying multiple anti-seizure medications, Emma continued to experience frequent seizures that disrupted her daily life. After hearing about the potential benefits of CBD for epilepsy, Emma's parents decided to explore CBD oil as an adjunctive therapy. Remarkably, Emma's seizure frequency decreased significantly, allowing her to enjoy a more normal childhood and reducing the burden on her family.

Section 14.5: Sleep Improvement

James' Story (Canada):

James, a 55-year-old retiree from Toronto, struggled with insomnia for years, often lying awake for hours each night unable to fall asleep. Desperate for a solution, James turned to CBD as a natural sleep aid. After incorporating CBD gummies into his nightly routine, James experienced a dramatic improvement in his sleep quality. He now enjoys restful nights and wakes up feeling refreshed and rejuvenated, ready to tackle the day ahead.

Section 14.6: Inflammatory Conditions

Fatima's Story (United Arab Emirates):

Fatima, a 40-year-old woman living in Dubai, suffered from rheumatoid arthritis, a debilitating autoimmune condition that caused chronic joint pain and inflammation. Traditional medications provided limited relief and came with unpleasant side effects. Seeking a gentler alternative, Fatima began using CBD topical creams to target her inflamed joints. To her delight, the CBD cream provided soothing relief, reducing pain and stiffness without any adverse reactions.

Section 14.7: Conclusion

These real-life success stories and testimonials offer a glimpse into the transformative power of CBD in improving health and well-being for individuals worldwide. While every journey is unique, these accounts highlight the potential of CBD as a natural, versatile remedy for various health conditions, inspiring hope and resilience in those seeking relief.

Chapter 14 presents an in-depth exploration of success stories and testimonials from individuals worldwide who have experienced the positive effects of CBD on their health and well-being. These accounts provide valuable insights into the diverse applications of CBD and its potential to improve lives across different cultures and regions.

Chapter 15: Conclusion

Section 15.1: Summarizing Key Takeaways

Throughout this comprehensive journey into the world of CBD, we've uncovered a wealth of information about this versatile compound and its potential impact on health and wellness. Here, we summarize the key takeaways from our exploration:

- **CBD Basics:** CBD, or cannabidiol, is a natural compound derived from cannabis plants, renowned for its non-intoxicating properties and potential therapeutic effects on various health conditions.
- **Mechanisms of Action:** CBD interacts with the body's endocannabinoid system (ECS) and other neurotransmitter systems, modulating physiological processes and promoting homeostasis.
- **Health Benefits:** Research suggests that CBD may offer benefits for managing chronic pain, anxiety, depression, epilepsy, inflammation, sleep disorders, and other health conditions, providing relief and improving quality of life for many individuals.
- **Safety Considerations:** While CBD is generally well-tolerated, it's essential to be mindful of potential side effects, drug interactions, and quality control issues when selecting CBD products. Consulting with healthcare professionals and choosing high-quality products are crucial steps for ensuring safe and effective CBD use.
- **Future Directions:** The future of CBD holds promise for continued innovation, integration into modern healthcare practices, and global acceptance. Emerging trends such as nanoencapsulation technology, personalized medicine, and international research collaboration are shaping the trajectory of CBD's potential.

Section 15.2: The Role of CBD in Promoting Wellness

As we conclude our exploration of CBD, it's essential to reflect on its broader role in promoting wellness:

- **Holistic Approach:** CBD embodies a holistic approach to wellness, addressing the interconnectedness of mind, body, and spirit. By nurturing balance and harmony within the body's systems, CBD supports overall well-being and vitality.

- **Empowerment and Choice:** CBD empowers individuals to take an active role in their health and explore natural, alternative treatments. Through education, awareness, and informed decision-making, individuals can harness the therapeutic potential of CBD to enhance their quality of life.
- **Community and Advocacy:** The widespread adoption of CBD reflects a growing movement towards natural remedies, preventive healthcare, and patient-centered approaches. By fostering community engagement, advocacy, and responsible consumption, we can ensure that CBD continues to be a force for positive change in people's lives.

Section 15.3: Conclusion

In closing, our exploration of CBD has been a journey of discovery, enlightenment, and empowerment. From understanding its origins and mechanisms of action to exploring its diverse applications and potential benefits, we've gained invaluable insights into the multifaceted nature of this remarkable compound.

As we navigate the ever-changing landscape of health and wellness, let us carry forward the lessons learned from our exploration of CBD: the importance of knowledge, compassion, and resilience in our quest for optimal health and happiness. Whether as individuals, communities, or societies, let us continue to embrace the potential of CBD as a catalyst for positive transformation and well-being.

Thank you for joining us on this journey. May it inspire you to embark on your own path towards wellness, vitality, and fulfillment.

Chapter 15 concludes our exploration of CBD with a comprehensive summary of key takeaways, reflections on its role in promoting wellness, and a heartfelt message of gratitude and inspiration. As we bid farewell to this chapter, may it serve as a beacon of hope and empowerment for all who seek to unlock the potential of CBD in their lives.

Chapter 16: Resources and References

Section 16.1: Recommended Reading

1. The CBD Oil Miracle: Manage Pain, Improve Your Mood, Boost Your Brain, Fight Inflammation, Clear Your Skin, Strengthen Your Heart, and Sleep Better with the Healing Power of CBD Oil by Laura Lagano: This comprehensive guide offers insights into the therapeutic potential of CBD oil for various health conditions and wellness goals.
2. CBD: A Patient's Guide to Medicinal Cannabis: Healing without the High by Leonard Leinow and Juliana Birnbaum: Written by experts in the field, this book provides practical advice and evidence-based information on using CBD for medicinal purposes.
3. The Essential Guide to CBD: Everything You Need to Know About What It Helps, Where to Buy, and How to Take It by Max Lugavere: This user-friendly guide offers a wealth of information on CBD, including its health benefits, purchasing tips, and dosage recommendations.
4. CBD: What You Need to Know by Gregory L. Smith MD: Dr. Smith explores the science behind CBD, its potential therapeutic applications, and practical considerations for incorporating CBD into your wellness routine.
5. The Ultimate Guide to CBD: Explore the World of Cannabidiol by Jamie Evans: This comprehensive resource covers everything from CBD basics to advanced topics, offering insights into its health benefits, legal considerations, and product selection.

Section 16.2: Useful Websites and Organizations

1. Project CBD (www.projectcbd.org): Project CBD is a non-profit organization dedicated to promoting research, education, and advocacy around the therapeutic potential of CBD and cannabis. Their website offers a wealth of information, including articles, research summaries, and patient testimonials.
2. National Institutes of Health (NIH) - CBD and Cannabinoid Research (www.nih.gov/cbd-cannabinoid-research): The NIH is a leading authority on biomedical research, including studies related to CBD and cannabinoids. Their website provides access to a wide range of research articles, clinical trials, and resources for healthcare professionals and the public.

3. American Academy of Cannabinoid Medicine (AACM) (www.cannabinoidmedicine.org): The AACM is a professional organization dedicated to advancing the science and practice of cannabinoid medicine. Their website offers educational resources, clinical guidelines, and information on continuing medical education (CME) courses for healthcare providers.
4. Realm of Caring (www.realmofcaring.org): The Realm of Caring is a non-profit organization that provides support, education, and research initiatives for individuals and families interested in using cannabinoids for therapeutic purposes. Their website offers educational resources, patient testimonials, and access to their observational research database.
5. National Organization for the Reform of Marijuana Laws (NORML) (www.norml.org): NORML is a grassroots advocacy organization working to reform cannabis laws and promote responsible cannabis use. Their website provides updates on cannabis-related legislation, legal resources, and information on cannabis advocacy efforts.

Section 16.3: Conclusion

In this chapter, we've compiled a comprehensive list of resources and references to support your journey into the world of CBD. Whether you're seeking informative books, reliable websites, or reputable organizations, these resources offer valuable insights, research findings, and practical guidance for exploring the potential benefits of CBD and navigating the evolving landscape of cannabis-based medicine.

Chapter 16 serves as a valuable repository of resources and references for individuals seeking to deepen their understanding of CBD and cannabis-based medicine. From recommended reading materials to trusted websites and organizations, these resources offer a wealth of information and support for those interested in incorporating CBD into their wellness routines or exploring its therapeutic potential for various health conditions.

Appendices

Appendix A: Glossary of CBD Terminology

- **CBD (Cannabidiol):** A non-intoxicating cannabinoid found in cannabis plants, renowned for its potential therapeutic effects on various health conditions.
- **THC (Tetrahydrocannabinol):** The primary psychoactive compound in cannabis, responsible for the "high" associated with marijuana use.
- **Endocannabinoid System (ECS):** A complex network of receptors and neurotransmitters involved in regulating physiological processes such as mood, pain sensation, appetite, and immune function.
- **Full-Spectrum CBD:** CBD oil containing all compounds found naturally occurring in the cannabis plant, including cannabinoids, terpenes, and trace amounts of THC.
- **Broad-Spectrum CBD:** CBD oil containing multiple cannabinoids and terpenes found in the cannabis plant, but with THC removed.
- **CBD Isolate:** Pure CBD extract devoid of all other compounds found in the cannabis plant, including THC and other cannabinoids.
- **Bioavailability:** The rate and extent to which a substance is absorbed into the bloodstream and becomes available for systemic circulation.
- **Terpenes:** Aromatic compounds found in cannabis and other plants, responsible for the distinct flavors and aromas of different strains.
- **Entourage Effect:** The synergistic interaction between cannabinoids, terpenes, and other compounds found in cannabis, believed to enhance the therapeutic effects of CBD.

Appendix B: Quick Reference Guide for CBD Dosage

- **General Guidelines:** Start with a low dosage and gradually increase as needed.
- **CBD Oil:** Start with 10-20 mg per day and increase by 5 mg increments until desired effects are achieved.
- **CBD Capsules:** Start with 10-25 mg per day and adjust dosage based on individual response.
- **CBD Edibles:** Start with 5-10 mg per serving and monitor effects before increasing dosage.
- **CBD Topicals:** Apply a small amount to the affected area and massage gently into the skin as needed.

Appendix C: State and International CBD Regulations

- United States: CBD laws vary by state, with some states allowing the sale and use of hemp-derived CBD products with low THC content, while others have more restrictive regulations. Consult local laws and regulations for specific guidelines.
- Canada: Cannabis and CBD regulations are governed by federal law, with strict regulations on production, distribution, and sale. CBD products must be obtained from licensed producers and comply with Health Canada's guidelines.
- European Union: CBD regulations vary by country within the EU, with some countries allowing the sale and use of CBD products as dietary supplements, while others classify CBD as a novel food requiring authorization.
- International: CBD regulations vary widely across countries and regions, with some countries allowing the sale and use of CBD products for medical purposes, while others have stricter regulations or outright bans. Travelers should research local laws and regulations before carrying CBD products across borders.

Appendix D: Conclusion

These appendices serve as valuable resources for individuals seeking to deepen their understanding of CBD terminology, dosage guidelines, and regulatory considerations. Whether you're a novice exploring the world of CBD or a seasoned enthusiast navigating the complex landscape of cannabis laws, these appendices provide essential information to support your journey.

The Appendices section offers a comprehensive collection of resources, including a glossary of CBD terminology, a quick reference guide for CBD dosage, and an overview of state and international CBD regulations. These resources provide valuable information and guidance for individuals seeking to navigate the world of CBD with confidence and clarity.

Section: Sources of Reliable Information on CBD

When researching CBD, it's essential to rely on reputable sources to ensure accuracy and reliability. Below are some trusted sources of information on CBD:

Scientific Journals:

1. **Journal of Clinical Investigation:** Publishes original research articles and reviews on various aspects of clinical investigation, including studies on the therapeutic potential of CBD for different health conditions.
2. **Journal of Pain Research:** Focuses on research related to pain management, including studies evaluating the efficacy of CBD in alleviating chronic pain and neuropathic pain.
3. **Epilepsia:** Publishes research articles and clinical studies on epilepsy and seizure disorders, including investigations into the use of CBD as an adjunctive therapy for treatment-resistant epilepsy.
4. **Neurotherapeutics:** Covers research on the treatment of neurological disorders, including studies on the neuroprotective effects of CBD and its potential applications in conditions such as Alzheimer's disease and Parkinson's disease.

Government Agencies:

1. **National Institutes of Health (NIH):** The NIH is the primary agency for biomedical and public health research in the United States. The NIH's National Center for Complementary and Integrative Health (NCCIH) funds research on complementary and alternative therapies, including studies on CBD's potential health benefits.
2. **Food and Drug Administration (FDA):** The FDA regulates the manufacturing, marketing, and distribution of CBD products in the United States. The FDA's website provides information on the agency's regulatory approach to CBD and updates on CBD-related enforcement actions and warning letters.
3. **European Medicines Agency (EMA):** The EMA is responsible for regulating medicines in the European Union (EU). The EMA evaluates the safety and efficacy of medicinal products, including CBD-based medications, through the centralized marketing authorization procedure.

Academic Institutions:

1. **University Research Centers:** Many universities have research centers or institutes dedicated to studying cannabinoids and their potential therapeutic applications. Examples include the Center for Medicinal Cannabis Research (CMCR) at the University of California, San Diego, and the Lambert Initiative for Cannabinoid Therapeutics at the University of Sydney.
2. **Cannabinoid Research Programs:** Some academic institutions offer research programs or courses focused specifically on cannabinoids and their pharmacology, clinical applications, and public health implications. These programs provide valuable education and training opportunities for students and researchers interested in the field.

Healthcare Organizations:

1. **American Academy of Cannabinoid Medicine (AACM):** The AACM is a professional organization dedicated to advancing the science and practice of cannabinoid medicine. The AACM provides education, training, and advocacy for healthcare professionals interested in incorporating cannabinoids into clinical practice.
2. **American Epilepsy Society (AES):** The AES is a professional organization focused on advancing research and education in epilepsy. The AES provides resources and guidelines for healthcare providers on the use of CBD and other cannabinoids in epilepsy management.

These sources offer valuable insights into the current state of research, regulatory considerations, and clinical guidelines related to CBD. When exploring information on CBD, it's essential to critically evaluate sources and prioritize evidence-based information from trusted sources.

This section provides a comprehensive overview of reliable sources of information on CBD, including scientific journals, government agencies, academic institutions, and healthcare organizations. By consulting these sources, individuals can access evidence-based research, regulatory guidance, and clinical recommendations to inform their understanding of CBD and its potential applications in healthcare.

Dear Valued Readers,

We want to extend our heartfelt gratitude to each and every one of you who has purchased and embarked on the journey of exploring CBD for beginners with us. Your support and trust mean the world to us, and we are truly grateful for the opportunity to share this valuable information with you.

In this e-book, we set out to provide a comprehensive guide to CBD for beginners, covering everything from the basics of CBD to its potential benefits and applications in healthcare. We aimed to empower you with knowledge and insights to make informed decisions about incorporating CBD into your wellness routine and exploring its therapeutic potential.

We understand that navigating the world of CBD can be overwhelming, especially for beginners. That's why we endeavored to present the information in a clear, concise, and accessible manner, ensuring that you can easily grasp the fundamentals of CBD and its diverse applications.

Whether you're seeking relief from chronic pain, anxiety, insomnia, or other health concerns, we hope that the information provided in this e-book has been illuminating and empowering. Our goal is to equip you with the tools and resources you need to make informed choices about your health and well-being.

As you continue your journey with CBD, we encourage you to approach it with curiosity, open-mindedness, and a commitment to self-care. Remember to consult with healthcare professionals, conduct thorough research, and listen to your body's signals as you explore the potential benefits of CBD.

Once again, we want to express our deepest gratitude to you, our valued readers, for choosing to embark on this journey with us. Your feedback, questions, and experiences are invaluable to us, and we welcome them with open arms.

Wishing you health, happiness, and fulfillment on your CBD journey, Sincerely,

Instagram @RodneyLuisAquinoWriter

www.RODNEYLUISAQUINO.com

Special Thanks: Perez Lee @ www.MILEHIGHSFINEST.shop